VIRUSES KILLED by IMMUNE SYSTEMS !

Covid-19 and it's many cousin viruses are everywhere and will be forever (measles infections are back). Viruses do not disappear.

Note: We have many 'useful' viruses inside of us at all times. Doctors advise: "Keep Away from this Virus" but we cannot quarantine our whole lives;

FIGHT VIRUSES by making your

IMMUNE SYSTEM STRONG !

Viruses evolve every day and so does our Immune System. Our Immune System builds a 'library' of Anti-Viruses. We breath in viruses and build the Anti-Viruses, that 'vaccinates' us. This goes on inside us every day. We do not want to be around feverish, wheezing people, but if our system is stronger than their viruses, then we kill their viruses. If we are not stronger, we get an infection and must rest to fight it off.

" NO VACCINE has Ever been developed to fight airborne viruses, there has Never been an (effective) Cold Flu Vaccine" -ex-Harvard Virologist M.Haseltine. Laboratory-made vaccines can harm some people, a complicated subject, see pg 29.

Covid-19 is Not a virus that has super invading powers, it needs time to multiply, meanwhile our T-cells are building the Anti-Virus to kill it. However many of our Immune Systems are weak like they were in previous viral outbreaks. Even marathon runners or muscle-men can develop weak Immune Systems by exhausting themselves. Some common foods weaken our Immune System, you may not feel it right away.

Re-Infection After Recovery ? You CAN get sick again and you will if your Immune System gets 'run-down' again. You made the Anti-Virus for the first virus, not a new, different virus.

Continued Page 7

VIRUSES KILLED by IMMUNE SYSTEMS !

- **INFECTIONS:** Understand and Heal   Page 28

- **Flu, Mono, Strep, Cold:** How We Fight Them

- **Sore Throat ? Causes of Migraines & Rashes**

- **Fad Foods,** Fad Diets, Stupid Cures   Page 13

- **Osteoporosis / Arthritis / Milk & Calcium Myths**

- **Alzheimer's** Helped & Prevented   Page 146

- HIV, AIDS & CANCER: **New Information**

- STDs: a Logical Understanding and Approach

- **Best Vitamins, Minerals** ? You Are Wrong

- 5G, Cell Towers: Immunity & Brain Damage   84

- **Brain Food**; It's Not Fish & No Shellfish   <u>Page 19</u>

- Meat Makes Muscles, **Grains Grow Brains !**

- **Cheese OR Nuts**: Animal Fat OR Vegetable Fat

- **Insomnia** / Night Accidents   <u>Page 33</u>

- **Menstruation Without Pain** / Birth Control <u>Pg 40</u>

- Doctors & Nutritionists Are Often Wrong

- Prostate Fallacies / Urinary   <u>Page 50</u>

- Protein Excess   <u>Page 49</u>

- Diabetes: We All Have Diabetes   <u>Page 56</u>

- **Gluten** Explained On One Page

<u>List # 3 of 5 of Health, Food & Life Topics</u>

- Parenting / Abandonment / Kid's Discipline <u>Pg 61</u>

- Bi-polar / Autism / Dyslexia / Hyperactivity <u>Pg 67</u>

- Teens Cannot Drive & Talk / Sibling Power <u>Pg 69</u>

- Depression / Suicidal Thoughts Stopped <u>Pg 71</u>

- **Children's Brain Development Ideas**

- Breast Feeding Prevents Aids, HIV & Cancer

- Living Through Your Child; Who Is In Charge?

- Yoga & Meditation; Their Misunderstanding

- Chiropractic Damage, Injuries Best Treatment <u>86</u>

- Masculinization of Women, feminization of men

List # 4 of 5 of Health, Food & Life Topics

- Perfectionists / Tough Guys / Asking For Help <u>89</u>

- Alcoholism & Drug Addiction: NO EXCUSES !

- Sex Addiction / Love Addiction: NO EXCUSES 2 !

- Sick ? For Attention ?   <u>Page 102</u>

- Lying & Making Things Up & Not Knowing It

- Happy ? You Better Be !   <u>Page 105</u>

- Party Drugs, Psychedelics; Positive & Negative

- Past Lives Myths / Reincarnation Myths & DNA

- Religion & Responsibility   <u>Page 115</u>

- The Burial Scam Because Of The Fear Of Death

- Music & Dancing are Important For All Ages

- Positive Thoughts Can Lead To Negative Results

<u>List # 5 of 5 of Health, Food & Life Topics</u>

- FAD FOODS Part 2 Fad Diets   <u>Page 130</u>

- Warnings:?modern grammar? Punctuation, CAPS

- Summary of this First Draft

- Impossible Burger / Beyond Meat: CHEMICALS !

- Grain DEBATE, also 'Wheat Belly'   <u>Page 151</u>

- Topics by CATEGORY   <u>Page 140</u>

- Topics ALPHABETICALLY   <u>Page 143</u>

<u>IMMUNE SYSTEMS Kill VIRUSES</u>

Humans & All Mammals Receive The 'Building Blocks' Of The Immune System Through Breast Milk !

The Immune System 'Building Blocks' are Not found in soy or cow's milk, unless you are a cow. Without these 'Building Blocks' Our Immune System is Deficient. Notice the rise in Immune System diseases with the decline of breast feeding since the 1950's especially Cancer, HIV & AIDS, the biggest diseases in the first generations who were not breast fed. Let's learn how our Immune System works & then we will learn how to strengthen our Immune System naturally.

Our IMMUNE SYSTEM creates our 'Fighters' against Viruses.
Your Immune System components patrol the body looking for out-of-control bacteria & viruses & then they kill them. Your Immune System's 'Fighters' match your physical condition: if your blood is thick from clogging foods & your arteries have plaque* (cholesterol), then your blood cannot flow fast to get nutrients to your 'fighters'

If your Immune System does not receive Fresh Water, Fresh Air & Fresh Food's Minerals & Vitamins and Rest then you will become weak & the viruses will 'break out' or grow and you become sick as you fight them (a fever occurs to burn out viruses). Whatever name a doctor calls it, catch a 'cold', get the 'Flu', it's ALL the same problem: Immune System is weak from being run-down and a lack of fresh food's vitamins and minerals.

If Your Immune System is weaker than the virus then you will get sick & if you do not rest & fuel your immune system the virus will eventually kill you, So Eat Well and Rest !

IMMUNITY, NATURAL: Animals lick their wounds because they are ingesting the viruses that are invading the wound so that they can create an anti-virus. Ancient advice: " Eat the Hair of the dog that bit you ". The viruses in the dog's saliva are now in your dog bite wound and if you eat a hair from that dog with it's viruses our immune system analyzes it & creates the anti-virus & then sends it to the wound, Go White Blood Cells ! PS White Blood Cell count varies day-to-day, week to week, based on wether our system is run-down or rested and strong. Blood tests are Not always accurate and will vary with your physical condition, rest...

Mother's Milk contains the Immunity cells so there are 2 Very Different Types of Sick People:

Type 1) People NOT BREAST-FED who have fundamentally deficient immune systems.

Type 2) People who WERE BREAST-FED but who are chronically, seriously 'Run Down' in energy & proper cell nutrition.

Type 1) Suggestions: If anyone you know was not Breast-Fed make sure they read the Nutrition Chapters especially regarding Vitamins in Foods because they have an uphill battle health wise.

Type 2) Suggestions: Daily Life makes your system stronger or weaker as a result of the ratio of Resting to OverWorking. The strength of our Immune System changes every day based on what we do & consume (Water vs Sugar Drinks / Whole Foods vs Processed, Pulverized Food) so AIDS tests will vary from Week to Week based on Immune System strength* (The most well known example of wrong AIDS tests is Magic Johnson; when he tested positive for AIDS he was run down, then he started resting & eating well & he's doing great ! Lab tests can vary over weeks or month.

Diseases & the Immune System:

While I studied at UC Berkeley the Worlds Leading Viral Specialist, Prof. PETER DUESBERG discovered an error in the methodology of labeling AIDS ! The Billion Dollar Gov't-Funded AIDS Org. funding was threatened & blacklisted Prof. Duesberg from the medical world. Now, in 2020, his game-changing theory on the origins of diseases is finally winning serious attention. An unhealthy water supply will make people sick. AIDS is not a viral condition, it is a Health Condition.

A.I.D.S. =

A acquired through overwork, junk food, drugs, sugar

I immune system that is weak

D deficient of vitamins and minerals and oxygen from rest

S syndrome (they named it syndrome for scare effect)

= A.I.D.S.

AIDS became the new catch-all term to replace dreaded CANCER. AIDS is a made-up term for being 'Run-Down'.

Cancer, another catch-all, made-up medical term has been used to describe 100 different physical problems, all involving cells that were dying from poor life habits, bad environment & bad diet. Cancer used to be a scary word decades ago but as they learned bad lifestyles created cancers, a new disease replaced it, AIDS !

If you are exhausted you create less white blood cells that week AND A BLOOD TEST WILL SAY YOU HAVE AIDS THAT WEEK ! If you rested & ate well for a week & took the AIDS test again you would test Fine ! It is bogus testing methodology which gives more funding to the AIDS organizations & their big salaries. Hospitals can label a death whatever disease gets the most funding at that time, Ebola, SARS, AIDS etc.

Daily Life makes your system stronger or weaker as a result of the ratio of Resting & Eating Healthy to OverWorking and junk-food.

" A Healthy Person will Not get AIDS " - Dr. R. Jaffe

CANCER MISUNDERSTOOD using Coal Miner's Lung 'Cancer':

1) Coal Dust forms in their lungs & builds up sludge.

2) Gradually cells have so much dust they die.

3) Then the cell down the blood line from the dead cell dies also.

4) It looks like dead cells are growing but they are not, more are dying down the line from the initial coal dust sludge area.

5) Blood cannot get through the sludge to clean the area & gradually bacteria & viruses find & feed on the dead cells killed by the Coal Dust.

6) That is NOT CANCER, it is our normal viruses that we always have inside us growing because our white cells (our 'fighters') cannot get to the area because of the poor circulation from the coal dust sludge inside them. A virus or genetics did not cause the lung disease, it's the coal dust !

7) George B. Shaw & W. Reich had ideas like these in the 1920's but there is no profit for doctors in giving health advice.

Get those Miners out of the Mine, Breathing Fresh Air into their coal-dust lungs & Train Them as Solar Installers !

CANCER MYTHS: The National Cancer Institute (NCI) & IARC (Int'l Agency for Research in Cancer) announced:

90% of Cancer Cases Are Caused by Environmental Causes (bad air, bad water, bad food, stress, bad jobs like mining).

Only 10% of Cancer Cases are Hereditary, (ancestors with bad genetics, who got them mostly from their environment and food !)

" Cancer Research contains a conspiracy to hide natural cures, strong evidence of natural healing was & still is suppressed."
-US Senate Hearing

Cancer is not a virus to be radiated, the 'Cancer' condition is dead & dying cells caused by a lack of oxygen &/or healthy nutrition. Dead cells block nutrients from getting to living cells & then they die too; the 'cancer' is Not spreading, it is just more cells dying. Flush the body with fresh vegetable juices to clean out the dead cells & revive the malnourished ones !

Travel & Your Immune System: All government mandated travel shots must be received. Within the same country a different water district has different bacteria than your home water system. Try this: as soon as I arrive in a distant area I drink a small amount of the new area's tap water. Then I drink bottled water for the next 24 hours while my immune system analyzes & creates antibodies if there are any unknown germs in their water. After 24 hours I drink a glass of their local water. If I'm not feeling anything unusual on the 2nd day my immune system has most likely acclimated. Allow Your Immune System To Adapt Gradually To Bacteria / Viruses From New Regions.

THE 2 BIG FEMALE CANCER SCARES; BREAST & CERVICAL:

What causes cell blockage leading to loss of circulation & an abnormal build-up of cells & tissue (call it internal cellulite) ? A lifetime of Cheese & Egg Omelets with their clogging fat molecules builds up in the Breast & Cervical areas (cysts). The mastectomy that Angelina did rocked the world: Preventable ? I sure hope those diagnoses were right but there are class-action lawsuits because thousands of mastectomies were done & doctors admitted the X-ray machines were older & the 'shadow' on the X-ray was Not Cancer !

Could **Breast Cancer Exams** be done tactilely, no machines ? I think women should be feeling their own bodies for cysts. The preventative measure is to eliminate clogging / fatty foods, especially Ice Cream, Cheese & Milk, then there will be less cysts.

Big money medicine has been found to be money-driven even if some have good intentions. Pharmaceutical company kick-backs encourage doctors to prescribe pills & unnecessary surgeries.

CHEMO ?? Please talk to the millions who tried it. What % of chemo patients pass away too soon ? A Very High Number ! Try fresh vegetable juice-cleanse every day for weeks & notice how you feel better. Stop eating dairy fat & exercise & that will clean out the blocked areas (the cysts). If bad life habits & diet are continued the blockage will grow; so it looks like something is spreading on the x-ray but it is just the blockage area becoming more blocked !

" There is no book on women by a man that is not a stupendous compendium of posturing & imbecilities." -Mencken

<u>FAD FOODS, FAD DIETS, FAD CURES</u>

These are quick comments on these topics, this whole book addresses these subjects in more detail.

-BRAIN PILLS for Memory: from Jellyfish ? what a scam, page 22

-POMEGRANATE, COCONUT, INFUSED WATERS: Every fruit & food has its own vitamins & minerals but none are magical no matter which science lab they paid off. Apples, Grapes & Pears are just as Great as any Fad Fruit. (more in Fads part 2 page 136)

-WHEAT GRASS, SPROUTS, ALGAE, SPIRULINA, all have green chlorophyl which is good but drinking the juice of immature plants or weird stuff is a FAD created by the growers for profit. If your taste buds are not warped they tell you, usually by bitterness, when foods are not mature, not ready to be consumed.

-Carb CONFUSION: Books criticizing rice & wheat should criticize WHITE RICE & WHITE FLOUR, Chemicalized & Sugared causing bloating. WHOLE GRAINS still have the outer shell w/ roughage & the B-Complex for Brain Functions. see pages 8 & 152.

-KOMBUCHA: WIKI: "potential harms from drinking kombucha outweigh any unclear benefits, so it is not recommended for therapeutic purposes." Better Probiotics for Intestinal Flora: pickles, salads, sauerkraut, miso soup, Vegetables, Juices !

BEST FAD: KALE; Dark Leafy Greens give us so many nutrients; Calcium, Iron, Chlorophyll. Steamed or Boiled for 3 minutes is better for our stomach than Raw. See Osteoporosis section.

2nd BEST FAD: JUICES; Fresh Vitamin Influx. Green Vegetable juice is best but any juice is better than soda. Juices are concentrated so do not overdue but old people's cells could use daily fresh juice with Soil Water, Minerals & Chlorophyll:

-Cucumber
-Celery
-Kale
-Spinach
-Beet: strong minerals & natural sugar to sweeten

-PALEO / KETO ? Eat animal fats & organs like a caveman! ha! The revolt against carbos should have been aimed at FLOUR, Chemicalized & Sugared that clog us, not the healthy carbos in Whole Grains & Squashes. ps Cavemen only ate meat when they caught it, they ate mostly roots, vegetables, fruits & nuts; natural, not processed flour products.

-VITAMIN PILLS, SHAKES, POWDERS: These are Old, Dead Ingredients that cost pennies to make in laboratories. The high concentrations cause you to feel a boost like sugar or caffeine but the Side-Effects are happening inside you over the long-term. Drink Fresh Vegetable Juice instead. Much more pg 142.

(more FAD FOODS, STUPID DIETS Page 130)

<u>OSTEOPOROSIS / ARTHRITIS</u>

<u>MILK & CALCIUM MYTHS</u>

**Calcium In Cow Milk Is Not The Same Genetically
as The Calcium Needed By Humans from Green Vegetables.**

Cow's Milk leads to Deterioration of Human Bones.

Cheese, Milk & Egg Companies paid researches, the FDA & AMA to publish distorted lab-results to scare women about brittle bones and to buy milk, cheese & yogurt with their fake calcium reports.

**Bones Get Brittle & Joints Ache from a Lack of Lubrication, the
lubrication we received for millions of years from the
Mineralized Water found in Fresh Vegetables & Fruits.**

**CALCIUM's best source for humans is
Green Vegetable's Chlorophyl
which also gives our blood IRON & OXYGEN.**

Cow Milk Grows Baby Cows ! Cows are Stupid and Slow ! Human Brains need PHOSPHORUS which is NOT FOUND in Cow's Milk, no matter what scientist they paid off. We now have 3 generations of people who drank Cow Milk their whole lives; these people have become genetically modified into a new hybrid species. Human bone requirements are different than cows, cow milk drinkers have weaker bones, although bigger. ps Mammals Milk is made from their Blood, cow's milk is made from cow's blood, Moo !

Humans need the Calcium & Phosphorous from Green Leafy Vegetables after breast feeding is completed.

Human Calcium: the Green color in plants is CHLOROPHYL, which when digested turns into or transmutes into 2 things:

1) Green Chlorophyl turns into CALCIUM for BONES

2) Green Chlorophyl turns into IRON*, enters our blood & attracts OXYGEN when passing the lungs. Then our iron-rich, oxygen-rich blood pumps out to our brain, every organ & every cell !

3) PHOSFOROUS, important for human brains, is found in GREENS, NOT found in Cow's Milk.

Milk & Cheese sales are down as this info is spread so you see more advertising / brainwashing about animal milk. There are many animal milk substitutes (rice milk, almond milk, soy milk, etc) which are creamy, gunky foods also BUT do Not have the Animal Fat, Hormones, Steroids or Animal Genetics because most importantly, human organs & brains did not evolve from us eating Cow's Milk.

The best lubrication for our joints is what our bodies have produced for millions of years from eating Fresh Green Vegetables. Our ancestors only domesticated cows recently & even then had limited cow's milk, if they were rich enough to own a cow, so human bodies are not evolutionarily used to dairy.

**Eat Fresh Green Vegetables containing Fresh Vitamins
& You Will Not Have Bone Problems or Joint Pain !**

(unless you overdue physical activity, lift too much weight,
or have too much weight on your joints, etc)

Ice-Cream, Cheese, Milk: These foods clog our arteries & heart & take years to eliminate their fat molecules. LOW-FAT cow's milk still has clogging fat molecules. Cleaning your body from the gunk of Cheese, Milk & Eggs sludge takes time but every bite of vegetables helps the cleanse. Dietary changes may not be seen or felt right away but they are happening on the inside, one molecule at a time. Sometimes eruptions in the skin (pimples, rashes) occur from old sludge being pushed out through the skin, that is good & skin eruptions will stop. Drink fresh vegetable juices for cleansing.

COW MILK & CHEESE EVERY DAY IS NEW to human arteries since refrigeration & corporate dairy farms have made cow milk widespread with poor-quality milk with steroids & antibiotics. Our ancestors only had milk & cheese on special occasions, Not Every Meal. ps America had NO COWS until Columbus brought them with horses, pigs, animal-diseases & hard liquor.

ALL humans are Intolerant of other animal's milk but some genetic groups handle animal milk better, although they still having artery-clogging issues. 90% of the Chinese are Lactose-Intolerant of milk & cheese; their culture never relied on it in their diet.

Dairy Substitutes: Soy & Rice-Cream & Rice-Cheese have no animal fat but it is STILL a thick substance that still clogs us although they are easier to digest; plant based fats vs animal fats.

Seaweed, Sea-Vegetables Are Green Vegetables: Our Blood has 95% of the same ingredients as Sea Water; identical ionic & chemical composition proving we evolved from the sea. Therefore Sea-Vegetables (Seaweeds) are the plants which nourishes our blood best because the vitamin & mineral composition of the sea is what humans evolved in. Sushi has a layer of seaweed. Traditional Japanese families have UNPASTEURIZED MISO before Every Meal to put live bacteria in their intestines to increase food digestion. Research over 50 years since Nagasaki shows Miso helps cells clean radiation !

The Darker The Green Vegetable The More Chlorophyl It Has:

- Boil Or Steam Dark Leafy Greens until they are Not Bitter, 4 minutes ? sample every minute. some like raw but if they do not break down fully when chewed then that is rough on the stomach.

- Make Them Taste Good With Sauces & Oils !

KALE, the best of the leafy greens
SPINACH
GREEN CHARD
MUSTARD GREENS
LETTUCES, Dark Greens

Green Beans, Celery & Cucumbers are great Roughage to push that Rice or Meat through our intestines. Eat Green Vegetables everyday for a few months & you will feel like a new person, like the lively people we were before cow ranchers took over Africa, europe, and then the americas.

* **LIVER MYTH for IRON:** (repeated) Slaughterhouses had cow livers leftover & so they paid greedy scientists to put out distorted information about the quality of iron in cow's liver to get people to buy those unsold cow livers ! The liver is where the cow's lifetime of toxins are filtered & they get people to eat it, bastards. Green vegetables have given humans iron for millions of years.

BRAIN FOOD; It's Not Fish, It's Whole Grains

DO NOT EAT SHELLFISH

Cow & Chicken Companies Paid To Distort Nutritional Facts.

Meat, Cheese, Fish & Eggs have protein, fat and nutrients which the brain uses for energy but those are Not the B-Complex of Vitamins that Our Brains Use for Nervous System Communications.

**Brain Communication Nutrients, the B-Complex,
are best found in
OATMEAL & BROWN RICE
and All Whole Grains.**

Neurons of the Nervous System communicate with each other through neurotransmitters & the main ingredient in that communication is the B-Complex of Vitamins. The medical world knows the Brain needs the B-Complex; doctors still give injections or pills of the B-Complex for a short-term 'fix' for patients with NERVOUS SYSTEM DISORDERS.

Nervous System Disorders / Mental Problems are common because modern people stopped eating Oatmeal & Wheat & Brown Rice everyday as all humans did before meat became available daily. Mental Problems can be helped by feeding the brain whole grains with it's B-Complex of vitamins, not Chemicalized, Sugared, processed, pulverized breads & pastas. Your Brain & Body Cannot Run Well On Junk Food.

Whole Grains is the Main Food the World Has Been Eating for 13,000 Years. Every Race & Culture on the Planet is eating Whole Grains Right Now ! Brown Rice, Oats, Barley, Corn, Wheat, Millet, Not Chemicalized, Dead Flour. Our ancestors only ate Meat, Fish, Cheese, Milk & Eggs WHEN THEY COULD GET THEM, mostly special occasions. Our long intestines evolved from eating plants, meat-eaters short intestines evolved from digesting meat which rots quickly in the intestines. **Give Us This Day Our Daily Bread,** When that phrase was written bread was made Fresh that day from Whole Grains.

BRAINS ALSO NEED PHOSPHORUS FROM GREENS ! High Amounts of Phosphorus in Green Vegetables, ignore the Cow Company Fake-Paid-For Reports.

SHELLFISH eat the crap from the ocean floor, they are 90% Fat

Eat Free Swimming Fish that have Muscles & Swim:

- Salmon

- Tuna

- Swordfish (yes, some microscopic mercury, we try..)

Shellfish are even fattier than other animal fat because they do not move much, they super-clog your intestines & then those fat molecules stay in your blood, collect around your heart & clog your brain, for 7 Years !

" Lobster & Shrimp taste So Good ! " it's the BUTTER & SALT that tastes good. Eat Shellfish with no butter & salt and you will Gag !

<u>MEAT MAKES MUSCLES, GRAINS GROW BRAINS</u>

Meat's grease & fat taste great to many people but the meat industry paid researchers to lie that animal meat was essential for everyday living; meat is Not essential for humans to be strong.

10K & Triathlon Winners for 10 years have been Vegetarians & Vegans, they have better stamina, gazelles vs lions.

More Muscle Tissue Slows Blood Circulation. Extra Protein clogs our blood, causing skin tags, cysts, etc.

Early Vatican Law Banned Meat 100 Days per Year, they knew about too much animal fats.

MUSCLES need PROTEIN; Meat, Beans & Nuts

BRAINS need GRAINS; Best Source of B-Complex

Heart Attacks need Milk, Cheese & Eggs (ha !)

GRAINS GROW BRAINS: see pages 19 & 146

WOMEN and BEANS: Small quantity & chew 30 times per bite.

BEANS MAKE MUSCLES TOO ! But with No Animal Fat or Hormones. Because beans have no animal fat in them, they are easier to digest & therefore we use less energy digesting them. Therefore we get more protein energy from one serving of beans than one serving of meat because the meat takes more work to break down. Also, with every meat serving there are some little undigested fat & gristle particles that stay in the system & gather in our bloodstream & artery walls, especially bad close to our heart.

Beans must be chewed extra well so our saliva can start breaking them down. Cook Beans with Ham Or Whatever Flavors You Want & try different beans, they each have a unique flavor & their own protein & mineral components: Black, Pinto, Cajun Red, Lentils, White, Aduki; try them all.

Gas / Constipation: Having Gas 14 times a day is the normal byproduct of digesting all food, so relax. Extra bean gas comes from not fully cooking &/or chewing beans. BEANS MUST BE BOILED UNTIL THEY ARE SOFT, for hours.

CONSTIPATION means you have eaten heavy, thick, waterless foods. PRUNES are funny but have an ingredient that makes bowel movements happen fast. Try 3 Prunes and wait 24 hours. Eat other fruits & carrots, celery, cucumber, watery vegetables. Some Brown Rice or Oatmeal when you are starving. See PROSTATE section.

I understand the idea of taking in the energy of an animal by eating it, but a cow's energy ? mooo. I'd rather have Tuna's energy ! Most ancient 'dominator' cultures ate the flesh of their human enemies and deceased elders. PS Eating Animal Organs is disgusting, organs collect the animals toxins, yuk !

*** LIVER MYTH for IRON:** Slaughterhouses had cow livers leftover & so they paid greedy scientists to put out distorted information about the quality of iron in cow's liver to get people to buy those unsold cow livers ! The liver is where the cow's lifetime of toxins are filtered & they get people to eat it, bastards. Green vegetables have given humans iron for millions of years.

<u>CHEESE vs NUTS:</u>

<u>ANIMAL FAT vs VEGETABLE / PLANT FAT</u>

**Cheese & Milk Adds Flavor & Joy !
Too Much Cheese Clogs our Arteries & Brains & leads
to Heart Attacks & Alzheimer's.**

The Cow Companies Distorted Nutritional Facts by bribing Scientists, Congress & the FDA & Bought Advertising to Make People Think They Need Cheese, Milk, & Eggs Every Day to be strong & Made Them Taste Good By Adding Sugar & Salt !

New Research Shows the Body's Reaction from Cheese Is the Same as an Opioid-Type Serotonin kick or buzz, No Wonder We Love Cheese, it acts like a Drug inside Us !

Some genetic groups can handle animal milk better* but all humans are Lactose Intolerant of other animal's milk. Human milk is what has grown humans for millions of genetic years, our genetic ancestors consumed VERY LITTLE Cow's milk until recently, the era of heart disease ! Cow's Milk & Cheese have Cow genetics.

Plant Fats Digest Fully vs Animal Fats Clogging Arteries, so Enjoy Nuts & Avocados All You Want !

ARTERY PLAQUE: Plaque forms on our teeth from food gunk & we brush it off; vegetables 'brush' the plaque of cholesterol or animal fat 'off' the insides of our arteries. After cooking with cheese notice the 'hard gunk' on the bottom of the pan, that gunk settles inside our arteries !

Animal fats, are harder to break down than plant fats, especially as we get older & so fatty molecules are left in the blood & they attach to our organs**; Fatty, thick blood causes coagulation & cysts & menstrual issues. (see MENSTRUAL section) Nuts have Fats, But the powerful Cow Lobbyists distorted the info to say that Nut Fat is worse than Cow Fat ! Not True, Nuts digest fully right away.

EGGS are super protein but also super cholesterol, ok to eat a little for growing bodies or manual laborers but eggs are artery clogging for adults. Countries with low animal food consumption have low heart attack rates.

WATER CONTENT of Food: An easy gauge of the healthfulness of foods is their water content. We want our blood watery so it flows easily through the heart & arteries carrying oxygen & minerals. Vegetables=75% water VS pizza=0 water. Rice becomes 75% water while boiling in water.

There Are Many Cheese & Milk Substitutes that Taste Great, Why Eat Animal Fats that Clog Our Arteries ?

Live Enzymes vs Dead Food: Over-cooking kills the Enzymes which help digestion so our pancreas has to supply our own stored enzymes. Nutritionally-Trained Chefs always serve meals with a side of enzymes; Salad or Pickles. A lifetime of over-cooked foods leads to pancreas & other problems. Stir-Frying & Steaming vegetables keeps in more enzymes. Raw veggies, celery, salads & fermented foods gives our intestines extra enzymes, pickles, etc. Enzymes lose their energy quickly from oxygen exposure after being cut up so EAT VEGGIES FAST & FRESH !

FRUIT; Too Much Sugar ? NO. A Trained Nutritionist advised his clients to NOT eat LOCAL Fruit because of the Sugar content, ABSURD! Fruit's natural sugar is within a balanced complex of vitamins & minerals. Fruit is grown from the soil's minerals which have nourished us for millions of years. Tropical higher-sugar fruits are not in balance for colder climate people who are not used to tropical sugars but they are a great desert that is natural vs cookies.

Make Your Food TASTE GREAT;

- Boil Oatmeal in apple juice

- BOIL BROWN RICE adding tomato sauce, pesto, anything you want.

- Add lots of sauces to make the healthy food taste great. Some fats & oil is fine. After your taste buds stop being sugar-addicted you will soon enjoy the food's natural flavors.

- PS bad chefs DO NOT taste their food as it is being cooked, which is essential to making good tasting food, Taste as You Cook, if it tastes bad you can still fix it !

BEST VITAMINS & MINERALS ? YOU'RE WRONG

Our Blood has Exactly the same components as Sea Water, We Evolved in the Sea !

Sea Vegetables or Sea Weeds grow in Sea Water so their mineral composition is what our Blood was Made from ! Their unique vitamin make-up cannot be found in land vegetables.

Sushi has Seaweed; that black sheet in Sushi is Seaweed & Sea-Vegetables are the little green pieces in the Miso Soup.

Best & Cheapest Vitamin & Mineral Source: SEAWEED or SEA-VEGETABLES !

Seaweeds or Sea-Vegetables, dried or in pill form, has better natural vitamins than any other vitamin pill; & only $ 5 (Five Dollars). My fave is dried kombu (less fishy). You can put a small piece in everything you cook for extra vitamins. Yes, the pill is old, dried ingredients but if that is the only way we can get Sea-Vitamins, which are not the same found in land vegetables, then Go

Seaweeds or Sea-Vegetables are also GREEN VEGETABLES with the Chlorophyl all Living Things Need !

Where do VITAMIN PILLS come from ? They are made by distilling & freeze-drying the Fresh Vegetables & Whole Grains we are supposed to be eating fresh. The Vitamin Pill is their Old Dust ! You are Paying for Old Dust !

OVERDOSING ON STORE-BOUGHT VITAMINS: For millions of years what we ate changed or transmuted into the vitamins & minerals our bodies needed. People who ingest factory vitamins signal to the body that it does not need to keep making our own vitamins (because it's coming from the pill) so our natural vitamin producing ability atrophies, gets weaker. If you want an extra dose of vitamins Drink Fresh-Squeezed Green Vegetable Juice !

Also, the stronger the dose of vitamins the more side effects; the body reacts to the overdose by making the counter-substances to balance out the extreme you have ingested, thus USING OUR BODIES' VITAMINS TO COUNTERACT the PILL OVERDOSE; Net effect; LOSS of Vitamins ! All store-bought pills have too much of that vitamin, a dose that is extreme for our body to process.

VITAMIN FALSE BOOST: You may feel a 'surge of energy' from a vitamin pill but that is usually an ingredient not listed or the overdose, it is like 'speed' to your system, a buzz that depletes your energy core & will have an energy come-down afterwards, like coffee. " Chinese companies found putting JET FUEL in the pills they sell to us ! " -CNN

**Even If We Only Get One Bite Of Vitamin-Rich Fresh Food,
That Little Bite Gives Our Immune System some Vitamins.**

STDS: A LOGICAL APPROACH

INFECTIONS   (see next page)

Infections occur when our Immune System is Weak !

If INFECTION IS SERIOUS go to urgent-care for a Prescription.

If We Are Well Fed and Well Rested Our Immune System Will Create The Antibodies To Kill whatever Viruses Enters Our Bodies !

Sexually Transmitted Viruses are not super bugs that defy physical laws. They have to enter an opening in the body & then they need time to settle in and then time to reproduce. Washing precludes or stops viruses from even entering.

After any exchange of bodily fluids, Wash w/ Soap asap. Ladies: douche or rinse out with anything available (vinegar, lemon juice, water, soap etc). The penis hole is not an opening that fluids enter but a virus left on the penis overnight may burrow into the skin so always Wash Right Away. The hands have no openings but wash them before and after touching any body opening, standard hygiene.

A great example of how viruses are Not superbugs: hawaiian leper colony missionaries worked for years without contracting leprosy because they washed after exposure and they had strong immune systems from eating well & living well in the hawaii sun.

SEX WISDOM from the Ancients: The old courtship rules delaying intercourse gave viruses exchanged during kissing a chance to enter the other's body so their white blood cells could have time to create the anti-bodies to the other lover's unique compliment of viruses, the invaders. This is the same procedure as vaccinations; exposure to a small amount to allow time for anti-body creation.

VACCINATIONS: The problems seem to come from added Preservatives & too large a dose. Get advice from several Professionals, According to your genetics, your family background. Get One-on-One Guidance

Viruses need a wet place to live. Viruses are trying to find a home and grow. If our Immune System gets weak and cannot fight invading viruses than an infection will occur. Taking an antibiotic for a minor infection also kills good stomach bacteria so it is better to rest & eat fresh foods to make our immune system strong again.

The Sun and Viruses: The Sun dries up a skin-surface infection so more invading viruses have no wet place to land. Then our internal 'fighters' kill the viruses that invaded when the infection was open, we cover wounds to keep viruses out. The radiation of the Sun also activates our entire system and gives life force to all living things, get some Sun every day, 15 minutes is a minimum.

In Summary: if a virus is living in a puddle, the Sun will Not kill it until the puddle dries up and the virus has no more host or home to live in.

Echinacea & Goldenseal for Minor Infections: Echinacea boosts immune systems w/ different vitamins & minerals than we get in our daily food. Goldenseal has antibiotic effects. $5. in Supermarkets in powder capsules or liquid**(below) You can take 3 doses PER DAY for One or Two Weeks or until sore or minor infection heals. You can Not overdose or take too much as they are natural herbs, not man-made chemicals.

**Yes, the echinacea pill is dried vitamins & minerals but for an infection we compromise our fresh food preference (unless you can get fresh echinacea & boil it.) We're taking the echinacea pill for an extra mineral boost but it's not extreme vitamin doses.

If you cannot get fresh food the vitamin & mineral pills are better than no fresh foods. After years of junk-food, large doses of vitamins may be needed by the cells, Fresh Juices is the best source !

<u>INSOMNIA / NIGHT-SHIFT ACCIDENTS / DREAMS</u>

A Lot of People Have Trouble Sleeping, You are Not Alone !

8 Hour Sleep is Not the Norm, 6 or 4 Hours is more common.

Modern Life has become hectic with so many details compared to 500 years ago before electricity, of course we all have trouble turning off our billion neuron brains !

There are many writings from the middle ages speaking of the 2nd Sleep: After falling asleep after dinner, going down with the sun, people woke in the middle of the night, read or had sex & then had a 2nd Sleep, another 4 hours. This is not unusual or unhealthy. Notice animal sleep patterns; 3-4 hours.

If the muscles & brain are not working hard they need less sleep. Athletes & physical laborers need more sleep, as much as 12 hours. Their brain may get rested but their muscles need more time to replenish so their muscles tell the brain to keep dreaming. Teenagers' developing brains & bodies during puberty need more sleep; older adults with less active lives sleep less, so relaxxxx & get some interesting books.

Try this QUICK IDEA before sleep pills with their side-effects: THIS SOUNDS TOO SIMPLE TO BE WORTH ANYTHING BUT TRY IT ! Take 20 Long, Deep Inhales through your nose and fully exhale. We have trouble sleeping because our brain is thinking too many thoughts, visualize clouds or ocean waves. If life's details come into your mind, say to your brain "STOP THINKING THOSE DETAILS" and go back to visualizing ocean wavesszzzzz and you will feel drowsy....relaxxxxxx..... sleep will come....

Most Accidents occur at Night: People do not feel the gravitational pull of the Moon but the ocean's tides show it. From 10pm-3am we may not feel the Sun's Gravity from the other side of the world but it is pulling our muscles down & causing accidents. Night work is against our billion year sleeping pattern, we're not night owls! Sleep before midnight is the most beneficial, one hour's sleep before midnight is worth two hour's sleep after midnight, so go to bed early!

5 Minute Naps are amazing in how they rejuvenate us. It is not logical; how can the brain 're-boot' from 5 minutes of sleep while 5 minutes of deep breathing does not have the same effect ? Sleep is a Magical Brain Function. But even if you do not fall fully asleep, deep breathing still replenishes. Sleep is deep breathing with little energy output. So even if you are not fully asleep, just relaxing the muscles & mind & breathing oxygen into the muscles & brain, even if for 5 minutes, will make you feel refreshed.

2 Main Functions of Sleep / Why We Need More Sleep & Rest:

1) During Sleep our Brain 'Burns' new information into memory cells. Lack of Sleep = Poor Memory.

2) Oxygenation of Muscles, Organs & Brain through deep breathing & nutrient replenishment while muscle output is minimal. *Brain work uses more fuel / stored glycogen than normal physical activity so concentrating a lot depletes our systems faster than walking. Do not think because you have not physically exerted that your nervous system does not need rest, it does.

Sleep Aids:

-Sleeping Pills: Dangerous ! Sleep-Walking or Driving ! long term side-effects; Do Not Take Pills.

-Alcohol for Sleep: Beer, made from grains, is a great sleep aid.

-# 1 Insomnia Natural Cure: Marijuana, Indica; Follow State Laws ! The Chinese have documented marijuana benefits for 5,000 Years (Malaria, Rheumatism, Insomnia). After an initial 'energy buzz' comes drowsiness & sleep. Fun fact: 10,000 year old Chinese mummy had a 5 ft marijuana plant in his coffin / tomb.

" I Do Not Need Much Sleep " Fallacy: Some people brag about how they need little sleep. They are confusing feeling great after a short nap with the ability to go for a long period without a 2nd nap. Do not think you are superman even if you are above average. No matter how smart you are, lack of sleep will cause nervous system malfunctions; unclear thinking, thinking that you are lucid, lack of grasp of reality, mental instability, even psychosis; Just Close Your Eyes & take a deep breath for a minute, ok to take a cat nap, or longer if your body wants, sometimes we may want a nap 2 hours after our last sleep, body rhythms vary, realxxxx & zzzzzzz...

People Who Prefer To Sleep More Than Being Awake: These people say that they do not enjoy dealing with life, people, they prefer sleeping. Solution: Develop Better Brain Coping Abilities. Whole Fresh Grains makes our Brains Work Better! However people with serious health conditions may need long amounts of sleep to recover, the way a coma can heal.

Sleep Apnea; What a Scam ! Yes, sleep patterns can be interrupted by breathing disruptions; we cough, we hold our breath during a dream; this does not mean we have a condition that needs a breathing machine !

Dreams: Neurophysiology classes at UC Berkeley introduced 3 Dream Theories:

1) My Favorite: After the Brain has cataloged new info & then rested it usually has to wait for the muscles to finish rejuvenating so the Brain creates 'stories' / dreams to keep itself 'entertained' while it waits for the muscles to finish recharging.

2) ASIAN DREAM THEORY: remembering dreams is a sign of a troubled system, it can be physical indigestion or unresolved mental issues. " Dreams; the angel of indigestion "-Mark Twain

3) HOPI & AUSSIE DREAM THEORY: Dreams are a foretelling of the future, similar to zen idea of circular time, meaning all events have already occurred; a difficult concept for western linear minds. IF the Hopis & Aborigines' dreams foretold the future why didn't they foretell the coming of the white man and destruction of their cultures ?

Sometimes our dreams have specific details of real things in our lives; I think they are the details we have in our memories & are not a premonition of a future. Couldn't a dream of something that does happen just be a dream that coincidentally came true ? There are many unexplained dream incidents, the brain's abilities are complex.

Resting Is Recharging & Healing: Do not feel guilty to say you have to rest or have been resting, it is not a sign of weakness to need to rest, it is a sign that you understand & respect your body's limits. No one can do everything, prioritize your time to include rest. It takes time to get run down & it takes time to get strong....REST as much as possible; lions & most animals rest 18 hours a day.

Brain Evolution & Sleep Problems: Our brains have evolved to be very big for our body size. Our oversize brains often think too much so trouble sleeping is not just you, it's a result of our evolution. Quiet the many sections of the brain, focus on inhaling through the nose & humming with the exhale.

PARALYSIS DURING SLEEP: Muscles become paralyzed during dreaming ! This muscle paralysis is programmed into our brains from the millions of years our primate ancestors slept in trees. When we were primates, if we moved during dreaming we fell out of the tree, this genetic adaptation has stayed with us through evolution. Sometimes we may wake & our muscles are still paralyzed, or we can be in a dream & cannot move in the dream, we try to move but cannot ! Relaxxxx, your system is working correctly & your muscles will relax, but it is scary during that 60 seconds of paralysis that we feel sometimes,

<u>SORE THROAT, MIGRAINES, RASHES, ALLERGIES:</u>
<u>Healed Naturally</u>

The Throat Is Our Body's Water Gauge. If Our Body Is Out Of Water Our Throat Becomes Dried Out.

There is NO man-made substitute for WATER !

People will take a cough drop or drink a soda but they USE OUR BODY's WATER to BREAK THEM DOWN so we end up thirstier day by day until we get sick.

Every action we do, every breath we take, uses up some of our internal water & every substance we consume uses water from our system to metabolize or break it down.

An Extremely de-hydrated person may need several gallons of water to replenish their H20 fully, keep drinking until your throat is not scratchy or sore to swallow. It may seem like a lot of water but if the throat is sore keep drinking, glass by glass.

Migraines & Headaches: Chronic or Occasional:

CHRONIC, DAILY HEADACHES is a bad sign showing deep, nutritional &/or psychological imbalance BUT Good News: Every meal your blood & constitution changes a little bit. Depending on background, change may take time BUT start today, contact a professional asap & read this whole book.

HEADACHES come from excesses, our brain is telling us TO STOP ! Think about what pattern you are doing excessively before taking pills or aspirin with their internal side-effects. A pill will block your pain receptors but your brain or body will still be out of sync;

1 **Cause of Headaches:** Lack of Oxygen in the Brain, Breathe In !

Other Headache Causes:
-Cold ?
-Hungry ?
-Too much coffee ?
-Excess Sugar ?
-Energy Drinks with sugar & caffein ?
-Medication's side-effects, sleeping pills ?
-Lack of sleep ?
-Tight high-heels ?
-Excess Anything ?

Overthinking causes shallow breathing or holding one's breath so the brain becomes knotted in concentration, a tight ball of stress. Hectic, caffeinated lives do not allow time for Breathing. Breath deep 5 times & you will feel less tense. 20 Times & your tension headache should be gone. I have never gotten past 20 Deep Breaths without either falling asleep or remembering I had to do something !

Skin Rashes, Breakouts, Sores:

Painful, Oozing Rashes may be a Viral Infection, go to Urgent Care & inquire about Anti-Viral Medication.

Normal rashes, pimples, etc can appear when we do not eliminate all our toxins in the bathroom. Toxins thrown off through the skin is good, your body is working, BUT Stop eating greasy junk food, sugar & cow products ! Lotions & Salves can alleviate temporarily but if there are rashes the blood is filled with grease, fat, sugars. Quick Blood Cleansers are Vegetable Juices & Soups, especially Miso Soup from any sushi restaurant but daily diet must be improved for lasting health.

Eat Healthy Food Every Day & You Will Become Healthy !

Allergies: Most allergies today are a result of our junk-food blood, with it's toxins / impurities, reacting to normal pollen, dust, etc. Eating healthier is the cure. As your healthy food turns into your new blood it will not react to normal life. There are genetic allergies according to one's background (wheat for some ?).

Genetic allergies are individual & come from blood type, immune system background, etc. They can be changed over years of eating differently BUT a reaction to bad foods (shellfish, liver, organs, etc) is not because of specific genetics, everyone has a bad reaction internally to bad foods even if they do not notice it right away.

Boring Water ? If someone's taste buds are still conditioned by our sugar childhoods & the only way they will drink water is to add flavor, then do it. If you must, add juice or tea bag, esp chamomile. As a person cleans out fresh water will taste wonderful on it's own.

Cough Drops can be useful if a glass of water is not available but the concentrated cough drop uses Your Body's Water to dissolve it so drink an extra glass of water to dissolve the cough drop.

EIGHT GLASSES of water A DAY ? WRONG. That old idea has been proven wrong by new science; the liver is like a sponge & too much water puffs it up so it can not secrete toxins well. HOWEVER, if a person is Very dehydrated (too much sugar or salt or both !) they may need Gallons of water to replenish.

Only Drink When You Are Thirsty.

COLD, FLU, MONO, STREP ?

Whatever a doctor calls it, it is the same problem;

YOUR IMMUNE SYSTEM HAS BECOME WEAK !

Viruses & Bacteria get out of control inside of us because our Immune System is too Weak from a lack of Rest & Proper Nutrition to keep the bacteria in check. When the body gets 'sick', 'breaks down', that is the body's way of saying: " I cannot go on, you are working me too hard: you are not treating me well." See Immune System pg 56.

Cold Pills with amphetamines or speed, gives you an energy boost but it steals this energy from your reserves. If you are run-down with no energy reserve, then your body will tear down tissue from your internal organs to get that energy, even your brain.

Antibiotics & chemo do kill viruses BUT they also kill the good bacteria & viruses residing in the stomach which breaks down nutrients in our food. After antibiotics food goes through us without complete vitamin or energy absorption.

Pills leech minerals from our system to break down the pill's ingredients & counter it's Side-Effects.

Getting sick & tired does not occur overnight; the symptoms can appear overnight but the internal run-down has been going on for a long time; positive results can take time from lifestyle changes. Every beat of your heart is sending blood cleaning your arteries (or clogging them with more Fat) The older & weaker the system then the longer rejuvenation takes & the slower the results are seen but our bodies are amazingly reactive.

Mucous Membranes: A fever burns out toxins so get that mucous out; do not stop your mucous flow with drugs. Mucous forms every time we ingest a substance that our body has a negative reaction to. Hot Spices is an easy example. So you can track your body's reaction to food by tracking your subsequent mucous production.

Turning off the energy-using brain: Mental work uses up more calories than light manual labor, so turning off the brain allows more rest. Emotions burn a lot of calories too. Worrying, Anger & Complaining tightens us, restricts blood flow & makes our system less healthy. Positive thoughts release tension; take 5 Deep Breaths of Air.

Only a few hundred years ago Chemicalized, Bleached, Processed, Pulverized foods were invented & that's when all the modern diseases started; polio, MS, etc. Health problems also come from overeating animal fats from cow & chicken companies.

A Person's Constitution is what their Ancestors Ate & Did.

**Your Future Will Be What You Eat &
How You Treat Yourself.**

<u>MENSTRUATION WITHOUT PAIN</u>

<u>BIRTH CONTROL EXPLAINED</u>

Ovulation, Periods & the 28 Day Lunar Cycle

It's been shocking to me the large number of women who do not understand the basics of their menstrual / ovulation cycle. (below)

The pain of menstruation is thick blood trying to escape through thin capillaries, ouch. The food we eat becomes our blood within 24 hours. If we eat thick, fatty, greasy food then our blood becomes thick & does not go through our veins as easily, causing high blood pressure leading to pain.

Menstrual Or Migraine Pain Is Not Inevitable !

Blood viscosity or thickness changes from every bite we eat, molecule by molecule. The more 'watery' your blood is the easier it travels through arteries & capillaries. Vegetables & Fruits are 75% water. Rice absorbs 75% water while it boils. The planet surface is 75% water. We Humans & all Animals are 75% water; well, we are if we are not eating thick, fatty, sludgy foods making our blood thick & sludgy so that it hurts as it tries to travel through the capillaries.

Food Plan For Less Menstrual Pain: Eat heavier foods for the first days of the cycle* & eat more vegetables & fruit leading up to the 'Event', that should be celebrated ! Plan your diet with your cycle & you will have less pain. Most 3rd world women have zero pain during their menstruation, try more fresh fruit & veggies.

Meat, Dairy, Cheese, Eggs, Pizza, etc have ZERO Water. If you want to have the pain of thick blood trying to go through your capillaries during menstruation then eat lots of cheese & eggs & yogurt & milk & ice cream ! or Discipline !

OVULATION: Tracking a female's 28 Day Cycle is the basis for preventing Pregnancy. Many women are sensitive enough to feel the little 'pinch' when the ovary releases the egg each month & 10 days later that egg can be fertilized. Women who are biologically 'in sync' with the moon have their periods like clockwork, it is something to strive for. In our modern crazy world we are under so much stress it is common to be off the moon's schedule. As women's lives become less stressful they will find their cycle will adjust to the moon. Women being around other women causes a 'cycle synching' to occur, as with all living things.

Birth Control; Natural: After a woman feels the 'pinch' of the ovary releasing the egg it takes 10 days for the egg to reach fertilization position in the uterus, so you can have 10 days of sex without pregnancy ! After menstruation the egg is gone so go full ahead until the next egg gets down to the uterus' fertilization position.

a BABY ? YOUNG PEOPLE READ THIS ! You do not fully realize the 24 hour a day, 5-10 Year commitment a pregnancy leads to. Birth Control is becoming harder to find in 2019 so to avoid a pregnancy a woman MUST track her monthly cycle so a missed period is noticed right away. (see NO CHILDREN in PARENTING section).

BIRTH CONTROL PILLS are effective but they are interfering with a woman's million year biological processes & have side effects that may not show up for years. Only use pills as a last option.
'Pulling Out' works BUT THAT IS RISKY ! Physical control must be practiced during teen years & is why athletes with control of their bodies are good at sex. Pre-Cum is lubricant without sperm however at some point they get mixed together so be careful; a baby is forever.

HORMONE REPLACEMENT THERAPIES; BEWARE; there will be negative side effects worse than the benefit, they are NOT what your system is capable of dealing with long term.

The menstrual cycle was found on carvings from 30,000 Years ago. Around 10,000 BC metal weapons & bigger populations led to male domination of the old Matriarchal Societies, hopefully that changes !

The Menstrual, Lunar Cycle: Over millions of years the gravity of the moon has pulled on all living things every day as it circles earth. The gravitational pull of the moon each day causes the ocean's tides & causes little 'tides' in all living water-based organisms. Also all water-based life is effected by the moon's 28 day cycle, in addition to the daily Sun's Gravity. Women's menstrual cycles evolved from the moon's 28 day gravity cycle. Full Moon Gravitational Energy causes Flowing. Males are not as aware of their monthly cycles & have less water to influence than women. Hectic lives & electricity cause body rhythms to get out of sync with nature so we modern people are not as lunar-synched as our ancient ancestors who had no electricity nor lived indoors.

MISCONCEPTION about CONCEPTION: When the many sperm reach the HUGE egg & knock on her door, the Egg analyses the genetic make-up of each sperm & The EGG CHOOSES the BEST SPERM of that batch!! They found during initial contact if the egg determines any genetic deficiency in the best sperm cell it has chosen it transmutes it's own gene to be stronger, to compensate for the sperm's gene weakness ! fascinating. So, Women Choose Between Us Men ! right from the beginning of our lives.

*** The Moon's Gravity & the Sun's Gravity are 2 unseen but strong forces on us. The basis of **Astrology** is the unseen effect of other planet's gravity pulling on our bodies' 75% water just as they pull on the ocean's water causing tides every day. Does the Sun affect you differently in summer & winter ? that is Astrology. Two simple examples of planetary cycles; 1) babies in the womb during summer heat become more active people than 2) babies gestating in winter. yes, alway exceptions from geography, genetics. Full Moons reflect to earth more sun energy & people act wilder with a little more sun energy, that is the physics of astrology. If you doubt planetary gravity you probably gestated in winter ! ha ! Mars & Venus have gravity too & Saturn is Huge !

WOMEN'S INTUITION: Intuition is not mystical. Intuition is being aware of the subtleties of human behavior; emotions, facial expressions & having a good memory of the past. Men who are more aware, more conscious, have good intuition also.

Blood is Life: Do not be afraid of having sex during menstruation, it's natural & blood is a Great Lubricant. This is the safest time for no condom, put down 2 big towels, put on some Barry White & Enjoy the,

MENSTRUATION CELEBRATION ! Full Moon Flush !

Menopause Occurs In Only 3 Mammals: Humans, Whales & Dolphins, Not Great Apes or Elephants. Why did this happen Evolutionarily ? Post-menopausal killer whales hunted & nurtured the group vs being pregnant & therefore that group had extra help. Evolutionarily the females who had menopause vs birthing older eggs, kept the group's genes stronger.

OLDER EGGS: Studies of children born to older mothers compared to their older siblings show the later-born child having less energy, being less robust. There are always exceptions so no need to argue individual cases.

FEELING YOUR EGG RELEASE: When a woman is in-touch with her body she will feel the little 'pinch' of her egg being released from her ovary to do the 10-Day journey to try & meet some sperm. The world is over-populated, let's hope it does not happen !

SEX BALANCE: Whichever parent's genetics are stronger at the time of conception, the baby becomes the opposite sex, evolution's balancing act. Proof; planet is 50% of each sex.

Ladies: You are killing your hair & fingernails. Stop following the magazines & movies for compliments from your co-workers. Coloring your hair will lead to becoming a balding 50 yr old woman. (dyes into scalp) Compliments to your nails are nice but they take away attention from your eyes and your other natural beauty !

+++

" There is no book on woman by a man that is not a stupendous compendium of posturing and imbecilities." -Mencken

jon here, I *cannot really* know female health issues but I am trying to help by addressing 2 big female health confusions. I welcome any corrections or positive suggestions. Instead of laboratory pills I am trying to suggest natural healing knowledge from the matriarchal era, before men took over from women in society, medicine and religion. Great book on the Female Goddess Cultures, especially 10,000 BC before there were too many people and not enough fertile land, back before men made bronze weapons: ' Chalice & the Blade ' by R. Eisler.

DOCTORS are often WRONG

Nutritionists are often WRONG

Lab Tests Are Often Wrong (Blood, Urine, X-Rays)

X-Ray shadow errors have caused 1000's of unneeded surgeries, class-action lawsuits are in the courts now.

In the 'POLITICS OF MEDICINE' class at USSC w/ Prof Domhoff we saw that Medical Books were published by the Pharmaceutical Companies advising doctors to prescribe their drugs ! The doctor's get kickbacks (eg; paid vacations) if they prescribe a pill quota for their area; that is wrong & probably illegal.

Doctors trained from those books are trained from the perspective of PILLS & SURGERY. Even though many doctors have good intentions, if they are taught biased information their health advice to you will be biased towards the companies who paid for the research taught in the textbooks. Medicines made in Laboratories, scientists & doctors making money selling sick people pills.

People are raised to think that Doctors Are Like Priests With Infallible Knowledge like the Pope.

Wrong Surgeries & Wrong Pills From Wrong Diagnoses: A Blood Test is testing living organisms in your blood. Our blood changes everyday, every hour as the food & drinks we consume are digested each day & turned into new blood. Blood labs are busy places. Blood samples can sit unattended for hours while our blood sample changes with oxygen exposure. Also, a microscopic slide or lens may not have been cleaned 100%, analysis machine readings are not always correct & can vary with electrical surges.

WESTERN DOCTORS Make Money When We Are Sick,

CHINESE & SWISS DOCTORS are not paid if people are sick !

In China's State Rural Medical Plan the town doctor is paid a monthly stipend AS LONG AS EVERYONE IN THE VILLAGE WAS WELL. If a person becomes sick the doctor is penalized part of his salary until the villager was better. This made Chinese doctors get involved in keeping people healthy; " Your kids are eating sugar ! "

? PILLS & SURGERY ? Is that all Doctors Have ? Ever notice how it's only the rich or highly insured that are advised to have expensive surgeries ? (heart, kidney, liver). Specialists get kickbacks from recommending surgeries. If you have no insurance to pay the doctor than their advice is to live healthier. Pills made in laboratories have side effects that take decades to discover. Don't be a guinea pig of modern science, try natural plant cures that have been used for 10,000 years by cultures around the world. Herbal cures have 10,000 years of trial & error. Our bodies need Vitamins from Foods not chemicals from a laboratory !

How Many Doctors Talk To A Patient About Their Diet ?
There Is No Profit In Giving Diet Advice, They Sell Pills !

Ethics of Doctors: The kindly doctor in medicine only to help people is long gone. Even ethical doctors need to pay off school loans, kid's education, vacation house; most doctors & lawyers Only See Money ! They were trained by medical books published by Pharma-Pill Companies so they do not advise diet change, they advise pills or a medical procedure, that the doctor & hospital profit from.

<u>Medical Fallacies:</u>

(see FAD FOOD & CURES section also)

Biggest Medical Scam:

Pharmaceutical Co's naming new illnesses that need their pills

- **Breast cancer exams:** (see Cancer section) Is there anything wrong with self exams looking for cysts (blockages), mainly caused by dairy &/or lack of blood flow ? (google current lawsuits from misread breast exams that led to unneeded mastectomies)

- **RESTLESS LEG SYNDROME ?? ABSURD** Your legs are cramped from standing / sitting at your job all day, muscles twitch! relax & take a warm bath! Restless Penis Syndrome ? Is this the next medical excuse for Tiger Woods ?

- **Asthma Inhalers:** Modern people consuming so much dairy clogs lungs. Sedentary lifestyles also contribute to poor breathing. Medicines (stimulants, speed) are given to stimulate blood flow but until the problem is changed the condition will worsen as the medicine residues build up & further clog the areas.

- **SLEEP APNEA;** WHAT A DOCTOR'S SCAM ! No-One has died from this made-up disease. Yes, sleep patterns can be interrupted by breathing disruptions; we cough, we hold our breath during a dream; this does not mean we have a condition that needs a breathing machine !

- **Skin Cancer Scare:** Cosmetic companies have caused a neurotic fear of sunlight. Yes, too much sun's rays are harmful BUT humans NEED some sunlight to have a fully healthy system, at least 15 minutes / day. (see FAD FOODS 2 pg 142

- **Irritable Bowel Syndrome & Constipation;** Eat Fruit, Vegetables & Water to Flush Your Intestines! no medicines

- **ASPIRIN REGIMEN ?** People eat a high-fat diet & want aspirin to thin their fatty blood ? so they can keep eating fat ? Daily pills build up internally, all pills have side-effects. Aspirin, from willow trees, is for when you have mild pain, not daily consumption.

- **BLOOD THINNERS / HEART MEDICATION;** We are all overweight from eating fatty junk foods so taking these medications as an attempt to artificially reduce our cholesterol without stopping the eating of fatty junk foods is dangerous because of the pill's side effects & the continuing fatty blood condition. CNN 2019: Causes Brain Damage.

- **Children's behavioral medications** Every school shooter was prescribed prozac, Pharma pays to keep that out of the headlines. STOP feeding kids sugar-cereals & caffeine energy drinks & they will not need pills to cope. Better Education too.

- **PAIN RELIEVERS:** Overuse: 50% of Americans are addicted to pain relievers. Find the source of the pain & work to change the source of the pain. If the pain took years to develop the cure may not be quick, but steady, daily attention to changing the bad condition will succeed eventually, Be Patient....reduce pill dosage & frequencies to the minimum that you can until source of pain is fixed.

- **Chemo Therapy:** no one survives chemo long-term, drink fresh-squeezed vegetable juices every day for weeks before agreeing to chemo but if you eat healthier you will not reach the stage where you need chemo.

- **TV COMMERCIALS:** PLEASE do not fall for these million-dollar tv productions playing on people's emotions. ALL Pills / Injections have SIDE EFFECTS that can take years to be noticeable, like BRAIN NEURAL DAMAGE, Change Your Diet & Lifestyle, Don't take Pills !

- **DIABETES BODY MONITOR:** If a person is so unaware of their body's energy level without using a monitor, they need counseling about slowing down to feel themselves.

- **Psoriasis:** Skin eruptions from consuming junk food & eliminating junk food through the pores. See Rashes section

- **1925 Quack Cures:** "...thyroid extract, adrenaline, thymin, pituitrin, insulin with pick-me-ups of hormone stimulants, blood fortified with antibodies against infections by inoculations or vaccinations of infected bacteria and serum from Infected Animals, and fortified against old age by surgical extirpation of the reproductive ducts or weekly doses of monkey gland.." - George B. Shaw,1925, Sound Familiar ?

PROSTATE & URINARY FALLICIES

Greasy, Fatty Foods Cause Prostate & Intestinal Problems.

Needing ' To Go' Frequently & Urgently? Yes, that happens with age. But DO NOT take pills / drugs for these life changes, the PILLS have Side-Effects that will be worse for you in coming years.

PROSTATE EXAM ? Similar to the vagina, the inside of the rectum has ridges & bumps which are normal, however money-hungry doctors will say the bumps are 'suspicious' & need testing or removal. The doctor's magic finger can tell the small changes inside millions of colons because we are all identical ? absurd. If you have No Pain Why Are You Having a Stranger stick their finger in your butt ? Fear caused by medical scare tactics to have us pay them.

Even Conservative Jay Leno quoted this on TV from his doctors:

" If you have regular bowel movements & have no pain, you are fine, You Do Not Need a Prostate Exam ! "

PS Any insertion into the rectum subtly damages the cells of the area making future problems more likely ! Yes, anal cells can give pleasure but that does not mean we go in there, like the inside of the ear or nose, do not go in there !

PROSTATE PROBLEMS: We can develop constipation from clogging, dry, junk foods. Our anus' pores can get clogged & cysts can form (blocked pores). Hot Baths with Epson Salts & sitting on a heating pad will open pores & cysts. Our anus may become swollen but less junk food & fats & more watery fruit & vegetables will be cleaner to eliminate so irritation will diminish.

ELIMINATION EVERY DAY: A bowel movement every day is not a 'hoped for' occurrence, it is how all animals function. If you are Not eliminating daily your body has a problem ! Solution ? Watery foods will push food clogs through: try celery, cucumbers, carrots, local fruit (add your favorite dressings or sauces for flavor as you get tired of the same taste, yes, sauces are clogging so go easy on them).

SQUATTING & ELIMINATING: For millions of years humans & dogs & cats squatted when we eliminated & poor parts of the world still do. The compression of the intestines pushes crap out. When sitting on the toilet, putting the feet up on a stool achieves the squatting position. Allow yourself & your intestines to fully relax, no TV or radio, deep breath or read for a few minutes & allow your intestines to release fully.

CONSTIPATION: PRUNES may be funny but They Work, they are different than other fruits ! Prunes will get you going ! Eat 2, 3, 4 per day until you go ! There are so many products for constipation but unless they are live, fresh fruit or vegetables they are 'gunk' that has drugs. Do not take these 'potions' or pills with unknown chemical side-effects.

KIDNEY & LIVER: These are filters for the body's toxins, which is why you should Not eat these organs from animals, despite fake reports from meat companies.

URINARY MYTHS: Drinking too much liquids, even water, causes the kidney to swell & discharge less. Drink Only when thirsty. Urinating many times a day occurs as we age, relax & go !

'Anal' obsession with only eliminating in your home ? Holding back your elimination until you get home will have negative side effects in your prostate, go to the bathroom where you are, even in the bushes ! In 17th cent europe the aristocrats had toilets in the corner of the dining room & eliminated while still talking to others, no hang-ups for them like the Victorians, sexually screwed-up Victorians !

Elimination, Body Functions. Some people do not know:

-Urine should be beer colored;
too light = too much liquids
too dark = too many toxins, usually too heavy protein foods.

-Feces should float; if it sinks = too much heavy food; eat more vegetables & fruits, the foods with high water content.

-Gas: 14 times per day is normal

-Diarrhea can occur as we are eating more watery foods & cleaning out the bowels of the clogging flour junk & fats. Dry junk food can cause pain going past & through our sensitive cells. Give your system time to adapt to changes. If we eat clean, natural food like our million-year old ancestors did then our body will clean itself of all the crap TV has told us to eat; Sugar & Flour & Fat & Grease; Oh My !

PROTEIN EXCESS

We Do Not Need The Large Amount Of Meat The Cattle / Beef Industry & Their Faked Research Findings Tell Us.

Ideas about PROTEIN were created & spread by the Meat Industry to get people to eat meat everyday, even every meal. They paid for lab studies & distorted the findings, but Bacon Tastes Good ! duh, it's the salt & grease not the meat. Our bodies are not genetically used to the large amount of protein people have been eating since industrialized cattle farms made meat available daily.

10K, TRIATHALON, IRON MAN WINNERS over 20 years have been VEGAN / VEGETARIAN eating NO ANIMAL PROTEIN. Rhinoceros, Elephants & Water Buffalo are Vegetarians. The lion meat eater can only run in short sprints, not a long distance runner like the green grass eaters, like gazelles.

Excessive Protein: One of the ways excessive protein consumption can be seen is in moles, 'skin tags', etc. This is extra cell production from too much protein. Extra INTERNAL cell growth from too much protein is not seen but is occurring inside heavy protein consumers. This extra cell growth is Not Cancer but they call it that, it's ' Skin Growth from Excessive Protein '. see CANCER MYTHS section

BEANS & NUTS ARE THE BIG PLANT PROTEINS. Their are easier to break down giving more net energy AND the other health benefits over animal meat is the lack of animal Fats, Antibiotics & Steroids. Beans must be cooked until soft, boiled for hours.

Over the last 100,000 years our bodies received a normal amount of protein from everyday foods; rice, potatoes, squashes, etc*. The Cow & Chicken Industries do not want you to know this but there is normal protein for humans in practically all foods however there is no profit in selling rice, beans & nuts.

Some people think they need extra protein;

1) they say they are not as physically strong as they used to be
2) they say they are not as strong as others in the gym.

Answer to 1) Yes, we are not as strong as we used to be because we are older ! Get used to that for the rest of your life & quit having unrealistic expectations of yourself.

Answer to 2) Most people are caffeinated &/or on prescription pills (speed) & so their workout rate is 'pumped up' artificially. You cannot compare a normal healthy person's activity level to people who are 'jacked up'. Speed users eventually will have heart & other organ problems. Also, stamina & strength foundations are built in early childhood, they can be changed but it takes time so be patient with your body while it gradually becomes stronger.

You can boost your internal energy with extra vitamins, stimulants, etc BUT excess makes your system work extra to process & eliminate the excess. Adding stimulants when we lack stored glycogen / carbohydrate energy makes the body tear off some liver or organ tissue to react to the boosting stimulants…
OLD PEOPLE: boost your system with the extra vitamins more than young people, best from fresh vegetable juices.

It Is Not Necessary To Eat Meat To Be Healthy: Wrong facts are promoted by the cattle / meat industry. Energy comes from the sun into plants & then animals eat the plants & we eat the animals; go right to the sun-energy source & eat the plants !

HAIR QUALITY & FINGERNAIL STRENGTH are the manifestation of our protein health. Use them to monitor your protein intake. If they are growing your protein intake is fine. If they are growing too fast cut back on protein.

HAIR LOSS: A normal amount of hair comes out every time we wash it. If you have a lot of hair, more comes out. As we age we lose more hair, accept it BUT DO NOT take pills or creams with unknown side effects. Eat quality, natural protein for good hair in old age. Exceptions happen from genetics; some inherit grandpa's toxic food organs so their body breaks down sooner even if eating good food, too bad their ancestors ate poorly.

SAUSAGE, PROCESSED MEATS are mostly animal part leftovers; hooves, tails & what is on the slaughterhouse floor with the rat turds. hot dogs, sausage, pastrami, etc. are not digested properly & clogs our intestines, heart & blood.

In history most people could only kill or buy meat approx once a week, if that often. That is how often we should eat meat.

Intestines of Predators (dogs,etc) only 3 times body length so rapidly decaying meat can pass through quickly.
Intestines of <u>Plant-Eaters:</u> 10-12 times their body length.
<u>Humans:</u> intestinal tract 10-12 times their body length, 60 ft long !

Saliva of Predators (dogs,etc) : strong acid saliva with NO enzyme ptyalin to pre-digest grains
<u>Plant-Eaters:</u> alkaline saliva WITH ptyalin to pre-digest grains
<u>Humans:</u> alkaline saliva WITH ptyalin to pre-digest grains

We're not biologically programmed to go more than 4 hours without eating; we're foragers / gatherers always eating constantly; our intestines are 60 Feet long, always digesting, unlike meat-eaters.

Louis CK: " We overfed people never experience hunger; we get a feeling in our stomach of Not-Full which we equate as hunger but it is not. "

DIABETES:

WE ALL EAT TOO MUCH SUGAR, FLOUR & SALT

Pills & Injections: 50% Of The Country Is Taking Them ! STOP

Too Much Sugar Is The Cause Of Diabetes, the Sugar that Is Added To Every Food and The Cure Is Less Sugar !

Baby Food Companies know that babies become addicted to sugar & salt for their whole lives so they put sugar & salt into baby food !

1900: 4 pounds of sugar per-person consumed per year

75 Pounds a year now ! No wonder everyone is sick.

FORCE KIDS TO DRINK WATER ! (or no phone !)

ENERGY DRINKS & SODAS with 50 Teaspoons of SUGAR; not brown sugar, High Fructose Synthesized Sugar. Now we understand why kids are 'bouncin' off the walls'; what happened to Water, Water, WATER ! if kids hate water add a little fruit juice or sweetener but gradually their taste buds will acclimate to the clean, wonderfully refreshing taste of fresh Water.

Processed sugar has ZERO nutrients, so to 'break it down' in our intestines our own minerals are used. Putting sugar in our mouth therefore makes our immune system weaker immediately. It also kills our intestinal bacteria causing less nutrition.

SALT & SUGAR dehydrate us the most because of their high concentrations. They soak up a lot of our body's water & nutrients to break them down, to metabolize, to assimilate them.

SALT corrodes metal, it does the same thing in the body. Small amount adds joy to life, too much adds death ! Ha. Soy Sauce is the natural salt alternative, but too much soy sauce is bad too !

High Blood Pressure:

Salt soaks up water & makes the blood thicker, making the heart pump harder to get the thicker blood through the veins. High Blood Pressure makes the physical system work harder, leaving less energy for thinking, causing less ability psychologically to deal with situations, we need a stable mental place. Thick foods (ice cream, milk, butter, etc) cause thick blood.

3 Quickest Blood Cleaners:

-Jewish Doctor: Chicken Soup / Matzo Ball Soup

-Asian Doctor: Miso Soup, UNPASTEURIZED (all sushi restaurants have Miso). The Miso bacteria is alive so do not boil.

-Natural-Path: Juices, Fresh Vegetable, Green

What you eat & drink becomes your blood in 24 hours, drink in Vitamins & Minerals into the blood through juices, pushing the old toxins, fats, out of the blood - spend money buying Health for Yourself instead of on medical bills, drink any or all of the above daily until you are better.

Drug Use for 500 Years: Sugar, Nicotine & Caffeine ! We now have babies born whose parents, grandparents and great-grandparents were consuming these drugs every day, since these drugs were processed, that's 500 Years affecting our genes which warps fetal development and therefore people bodies and minds.

People Know They Need To Eat Better, But They Don't Do It; Develop Discipline !

Our blood changes every day from the food we eat eat so healthy, non-fat foods, whole grains, squashes & beans, with their long-lasting complex carbohydrate energy our cravings for quick-fix sugar will decrease. More importantly the B-Complex found in Whole Grains will fuel our Brain with steady energy for clearer, more stable thinking and actions.

Jon here: As I changed my diet in college, after a month I noticed that deserts became too sweet. My taste buds were becoming normalized back to where they were before sugar warped or addicted them. As my taste buds normalized Junk Food tasted like I was eating poison, and it was ! A poison of chemicals: high-fructose corn syrup, cane sugar and other poisons.

GLUTEN EXPLAINED on One Page

Gluten is Not the problem, it is FLOUR that causes intestinal clogging & the added chemicals cause rashes.

WORST: WHITE FLOUR; they BLEACH it to make it white and it is stripped of the fiber that is in the shell that helps us digest it.

BEST FLOUR: Fresh-Ground Whole-Grain with No Chemicals.

Gluten-Free Products made with FLOUR as Healthy ? absurd, a billion dollar scam ! Vegetables & Fruits have Zero Gluten, ha !

ALL FLOUR causes intestinal SLUDGE that needs to be pushed through our intestines with water based foods, Vegetables, Fruits & Rice are 75% water. ps Many people 'wolf-down' their food, slow down, try for 25 chews per bite to avoid intestinal blockage.

BLOATING, ALLERGIES, All DIGESTIVE PROBLEMS did not exist before Processed Foods were made 100 Years ago. Eat Brown Rice & Oatmeal for a few days, a few weeks, months; all conditions will improve. 3rd world villages do not have digestive problems.

Substitute for Pasta: SPAGHETTI SQUASH ! Boil for 20 minutes & the inside turns into strands like spaghetti but it's a vegetable with vitamins instead of old pasta flour clogging our intestines. Pour on tomato sauce, meat sauce, pesto or whatever you like ! You will think it's pasta but it's all vitamins & fiber ! Do not overcook.

<u>The MASCULINIZATION of WOMEN & the feminization of men</u>

STEROIDS & HORMONES in Our Food is the Cause.

Now that Burger Joints have announced in 2020 they will no longer be adding Steroids & Hormones we see the truth:

Cattle & Chicken Farms Have Been Adding Steroids & Hormones For Over 50 Years To The Feed Of Every Animal That Makes Egg, Milk, Cheese & Meat Products.

They inject them with extra doses of Hormones & Steroids to grow animals heavier for market. There are now several generations of people who have consumed STEROIDS & HORMONES their whole lives, every meal ! Now today's disruptive social behavior is better understood.

HORMONES & STEROIDS in all animal foods AFFECT SEXUALITY: We're getting genetically 'messed up'. Men are growing breasts, women's shoulders are getting bigger & more women are having trouble getting pregnant, we are genetically mutating. Natural sexual polarity is diminished from consuming hormones & steroids.

PS I am not discussing here social factors, this section is about CONSUMPTION OF HORMONES & STEROIDS from industrial farming of cattle, sheep & chickens which made these chemicals part of every meal; hormone & steroid consumption in every bite, for 50 years, two generations.

Worst animal-feed fact: A BIG Texas farm owner was seen by the FDA inspectors dumping CEMENT DUST in his cow's feed to make them heavier for sale! -Mother Jones (received slap on the wrist)

PARENTING / ABANDONMENT MYTHS

Kid's DISCIPLINE

**A Child Does Not Need Their Biological Parents
To Grow To Be Healthy & Happy.**

**The Day-To-Day Love & Appreciation That Helps A Child
Develop Emotional Self-Worth Can Come From Many Sources !**

All of us need love, but it can come from others outside the parents; a piglet is happy with the love from a duck mother. A parent can leave a family forever but as long as the children have someone who gives them love & is a good role model they can develop self-esteem & have a healthy psychological & emotional personality, they can even develop from books.

The love we receive from others should develop into Self-Love. When Self-Love becomes strong, we do not need constant love from others because we retain in our memories all the positive attention we received growing up & we learn to love ourselves, even with our faults. Self-love is not vanity or ego, it is accepting yourself as you are yet still working to improve our weaknesses.

PARENTING IS HARDER NOW: Before mass communication parents were the few adults children encountered so they were special. After mass media children would hear of super-heroes who made the parents look smaller, much harder to maintain parental respect & authority. Solution: from an early age educate the child to understand super-heroes are fictional & all adults have issues.

Discipline = Boundaries Of Behavior

YOUNG CHILDREN IN A HARNESS / LEASH: Until a child's Social Awareness is a deterrent to their negative behavior, a human child is still at the stage of being an untrained animal, they may hurt themselves/others. The mythology of human young being any different than other animal young is utopian thinking.

GREAT BOOK FOR PRE-TEEN & TEEN GIRLS: ' Girls & Sex ' by Peggy Orenstein & Charis Denison with empowering messages.

BABY SLEEPING ALONE: We all need time for our brains to relax. Some can relax with a baby in their arms & some cannot. No animal has ever let their babies sleep alone. The plan of letting the baby fall asleep with mother & then move to another room with monitor seems good. I worry that baby alone, crying, causes emotional issues ?

Spoiled Children / Adults: Young Children Are Animals. No matter how cute they are they need to be trained to be social just like all animals. Boundaries of behavior must be established early & fairly enforced. Without discipline children 'spoil', become self-centered, selfish, spoiled rotten; bad. Once spoiled, it is harder to discipline them back into good behavior so discipline early. They do not know to be good socially until they see the negative consequences of hurting others. A spoiled person may rebel if disciplined too harshly, try a gradual 'tightening of the boundaries of behavior'.

CAVITIES: I wish I had been shown pictures of cavities with explanations so I would have been scared into brushing & flossing. Seeing filmed car crashes scared me to become a safe driver !

" Fear of god (retribution) creates Kindness " -S.Parabola

Abuse OR Discipline ? If we view young children (1yrs to 3yrs ?) as having no social awareness similar to an animal's peeing on the rug, an appropriate gentle slap sends a training lesson. " If you Spank Lightly Once you may never have to do it again."-unknown. Excessive physical punishment is abuse & illegal, but not a gentle slap. As the child's social awareness grows other punishments can substitute but even the government has physical punishment as the ultimate arbiter of social behavior; jail. My father's discipline approach kept me acting good. If I had broken the rules I was made to stand with hand outstretched ready for a hand-slap. When I was younger, a hand slap hurt & made me remember why I received it. When I was older, I was made to stand with hand out for a slap, which was scary, while a discussion was held about my bad behavior & after I apologized & promised not to do it again, I was often dismissed without the slap. BUT that FEAR OF THE POTENTIAL SLAP kept me from repeating bad behavior. Every family & child is different & children's ages are factors.

PLEASING the PARENT: Placing guilt on a child to perform is not a healthy plan. Positive encouragement, with discipline boundaries spelled out, will always be better. Good parents should let their children know when they are making their parents happy, give children constant encouragement, and adults too !

Food: You Are In Charge, Not The Kid: Any parent that allows kids to have decisions regarding diet is not empowering their child, they are spoiling the child. Childish food choices will increase their future doctor bills for obesity & sugar addiction (diabetes). Children MUST EAT their Rice, Oatmeal, Green Vegetables & Fruit & AFTER that they can have a treat. In well trained families the Fruit IS the treat !

" True friendship shows when denying a friend something bad for them. Love will give something harmful if we listen to the other person's desires VS caring for their well-being." -Goethe

MONEY CAN CORRUPT FAMILY VALUES: Parents who want to keep their children innocent of the money game have a good intention but is is a misguided strategy and like a lack of education about sex can lead to future confusions. A lack of education retards the child's real-world learning, they will be less equipped in dealing with life.

VALUES respecting our family, community and all living things are the most important values, and must be taught to a child before they understand money. Money is simply a tool that can help our family values but respect for our fellow people is more important.

WRONG: " Money is the Root of All Evil ". Money's Bad Reputation comes from when people hurt others, themselves or nature to gain money, like polluting rivers.
GREED is the Root of All Evil, not money.

MONEY is just a symbol, it is the FREEDOM it buys that is valu-able. However, freedom can be achieved without money. Teach children about money transactions early and MAKE MONEY FUN ! with Bets ! & Buying Apple Stock !

Test Knowledge with Betting which Gives Validation & Esteem: Betting does not have to be for money. Yes, gambling & sugar can be addicting but addiction is stopped by Discipline. Small wagers or bets are fun & a clear, visible test of knowledge, which helps self-esteem. Bets can be for chores or anything a person wants or just keep score over time.

SPORTS FOR KIDS: Young children do not need trained sports teachers; it is better for the parent to throw the ball to their child; at a young age (up to 10 yrs), correct form is not the main goal. When I was a sports teacher I had closer bonds with my teen students than their parents did, not the best scenario but can have benefits if the parents are 'out of touch'.

When the parent is on the sideline watching a young child learn sports from a teacher with no involvement from the parent a bad subconscious message is sent that either what they are doing is not worth the parents participating or the parents are not competent at this simple activity.

Failure Is How We Learn, if we are smart enough to recognize the reason why we failed.

Instead of paying a coach, play with your kids and YOU make the Rules, good for parents too. Rules change according to age & ability & can change mid-game to correct imbalances in abilities. BUT, Parents ideally will not be playing with their kids because the kids will play with other kids ! They only need an adult when it gets to be too many kids. Parents should be playing with Other Parents !

TO HAVE CHILDREN OR NOT ? More parents are confessing in interviews that parenting was 10% Joy & 90% Pain-In-The-Ass. However, if a parent is immature then raising a child can help the parent mature along with the child & can be more fun than loneliness. Having No children escapes the biological imperative & the societally-induced psychological and emotional directives. Also good for the overpopulation problem. Read D. Wallace ' On Deathbed..' re infants' needs & wives lost to motherhood. Also HL Mencken on Nietzsche on motherhood. (see Ego in Perfectionists section page 89)

" ..raising children has dangers & risks, full of strife & worry with few meager blessings. " -Democritus, read more from him on children

Childhood Myths: In   modern   times   a   myth   exists   of   an idyllic childhood, care free, all joy. This is a nice fantasy that only the rich can achieve, however, those rich children are often emotionally & psychologically stunted as they have no real-life experience. It is through wrestling with life & others that we strengthen ourselves & our mental, emotional & physical muscles.

Get Kids Off TV: Make Something In the Real World; Whatever age the kid is they can make something with their hands; an ashtray of mud ! puzzles train brains, hammer nails, clean house, think !

Working Children: It is normal & healthy for young kids to help the family with chores. Anyone receiving food, shelter from the family or community is expected to give back & this should be instilled if not learned naturally. If children are not expected to give back they develop an entitled attitude, their personalities become soft from lack of work, soft like fruit, Spoiled. When children work it develops not only their skills but their sense of self-worth, accomplishing things, becoming a mature person. After they do their chores, their off-time, play-time becomes much more valuable to them & a simple ball becomes the best toy in the world ! ps COLLEGE is NOT Necessary for most, more later.

Interrupting while Adults are Talking: Do Not allow interruptions, kids & animals need to be trained. Say to the child: " Please only interrupt adults talking if it is important. " Give kids a project to keep them busy but do not ignore them for long.

FRIEND vs ACQUAINTANCE: (some do not know the difference)

> - **Friend** is someone who will go out of their way to help you, do a favor for you, without expecting anything in return (if you are a good friend, person, YOU WILL do something of equal or greater value for them).

> - **Acquaintance** is someone who is not expected to go out of their way for you but acts friendly & may be willing to ' Trade Favors ', similar to a business deal.

Friend Boundaries: " I thought we were friends but the disrespectful way you have treated me changes that friendship & relationship. It may be repaired with your effort to repair it."

" Man is most nearly himself when he achieves the seriousness of a child at play." - Heraclitus

<u>BI-POLAR / AUTISM / DYSLEXIA / HYPERACTIVITY</u>

Drug Use for 500 Years: Sugar, Caffeine, Nicotine.

Brain damage has been occurring since these drugs were shipped to europe but Good News: Our Blood Changes every day from the food we eat & then our Blood Nourishes Our Brain back to good health.

Feed kids Oatmeal &/or Brown Rice Every Day for 30 Days & See the Difference !

Brain Communication Nutrients are found in OATMEAL & BROWN RICE and All Whole Grains. Meat, Cheese, Fish & Eggs have fat, protein and nutrients but those are Not the B-Complex that Our Brains Use for Nervous System Communications.

Our Nervous System's substance for communication since the cultivation of Grains 13,000 years ago has been the B-Complex of Vitamins found in Whole Grains. All Brain Functions will be improved if our brains are fueled with Fresh, Whole Grains. Oatmeal, Brown Rice, Corn, Wheat, Barley, etc. Not Chemicalized, Sugared bread, pasta or white rice.

**Give Kids Quality Food
Good Teachers
Good Books
Music Instruments
&
Watch Kids Self-Esteem & Love of Life Grow !**

DYSLEXIA: Reading involves eye muscles. Early TV-VIDEO-GAME-IPAD-COMPUTER viewing does cause atrophy, laziness of the EYE MUSCLES. Notice the rise in cases since the overuse of TVs & Computers. Hyper kids may be too 'antsy' for the slow art of reading & may be wrongly diagnosed as dyslexia when it may be sugar. Childhood needs to be spent outside playing with moving objects, like balls, which helps future driving skills by training hand-eye coordination.

Hyperactivity: Due To Excess Sugar, which companies have placed in ALL processed foods we eat every meal. Force Kids To Drink Plain Water & Oatmeal Every Day, or No Phone !

PRESCRIPTION DRUGS: Laboratory drugs are very strong, a behavioral drug can show immediate effects however there are always side effects to powerful drugs. Plants, Herbs, have helpful nutrients, chemicals, in a natural balance. Governments are funding studies on herbs because they work but also want to avoid the side-effect lawsuits from man-made pills.

Do not hesitate to scare children about future health problems from bad eating, just like we scare them to not touch a hot stove. Show kids the difficult parts of life with a conversation before & after. Teach them by showing them life's problems & make them repeat outloud what to avoid, what long-term issues caused the problems; like showing them pictures of Rotting Teeth from Not Brushing !

Don't ASK kids, TELL THEM:

" EAT YOUR OATMEAL

or NO phone "

<u>TEENS CANNOT DRIVE & TALK at the SAME TIME</u>
<u>SIBLING POWER</u>

The latest neuroscience shows that the Brain's Frontal Lobe, which controls the ability to do 2 things at once, does not fully mature until approx age 21-24 years with some older or never.

Teen Drivers (& adults too); Stop Telling Stories & Quit Turning Around to people in the back seat ! Human brains are not really designed for multi-tasking, no matter what magazines say. We can get away with doing 2 things at once if they are simple, but Not Driving & Talking. Let passengers do the talking as they pay attention too. Most Car Deaths are Teens.

-Drivers Must Always Focus Eyes Forward

-Passengers Need to be Told They are Extra Eyes For The Driver, Telling the Driver About Upcoming Traffic Issues, especially drowsy Truck Drivers.

SIBLING POWER: DEVELOPING A TEAM SPIRIT: The siblings together form a group, clan, clique. That is the power of a group, their inclusiveness, the sense of belonging to a bigger power than ourselves, but not be a sheep-follower to bad ideas, debate ideas.

Rule # 1: NEVER criticize a group member or team member or family member in front of outsiders ! However team members must be open to internal group suggestions for improvement; Help Each Other to Become Stronger !

Rule # 2: The Older must care for the younger & the younger must Respect the Older.

Rule # 3: All rules must be followed under threat of fair penalties.

DRIVING PATTERN CHANGES for Teens & You !

1) When Turning Left If traffic is busy GO AN EXTRA BLOCK & circle back to make it easier & safer, and maybe faster.

2) Wrong Way Drivers on Highways, some with NO HEADLIGHTS ! Be extra Alert at Night for these Idiots. All Passengers Need to be Told to Help the Driver & Pay Attention ! Passengers get killed when they do not pay attention, wait to Party until you get there safely, remind new drivers the car is a potential death machine.

3) Honking at a rude driver may distract them & make them crash, let them drive on safely & we'll teach them later.

ANGRY TEENAGERS: Hormones are raging; it's natural but channel emotions. Keep Kids Physically Active, Run them around until they are exhausted. No Energy- Sugar-Caffein drinks for teens.

SEX & TEENAGERS: Teens will engage in sexual antics. Forbidding them will not work. Fondling, kissing, dry-humping are not dangerous the way penetration is. Talk with kids or have someone trusted talk with them. Beware of sexual 'armoring'.

TEENAGERS & FAME: Teens Want Fame, what are they missing in their lives that makes them want fame ? Self-Confidence. Advertising keeps telling them they are inadequate so they will Buy. This is countered by Self-Confidence, Self-Love, which is Not sinful as the puritans want us to believe & join their cult. Teens & all of us need to Learn to Love Ourselves by working on becoming a good person & working on worthwhile skills that help our future in society.

"..our youth are uneducated & only have ordinary passions..insteas of discovering a rich worldview from the great men of the past today's youth are egoists, that is all they are taught " -Bloom

DEPRESSION and SUICIDAL THOUGHTS STOPPED !

Suicidal Thoughts ? Call Chat 800#'s, they are nice people ! Yes, life can become distressing or tedious or boring. Let's slow down & read this whole section, all 6 pages.

We are not made to live in cubicles in cities, running on caffeine, sugar & junk food; of course people are Depressed !

1 Cause of Depression: Tired Brain needs Sleep !

DEPRESSION is used to describe 2 different feelings:

1) Physically Depressed: Being tired or exhausted means our energy is depressed. If our body & brain power is low you do not have the energy to be 'UP' or 'Full of Life' or 'Happy' then you can say you are 'depressed' so Take a Nap & Eat ! Psychological issues can be addressed when we are well rested & well Fed.

2) Mentally Depressed: Modern Society has led to alienation & loneliness; *" Man is a unit of society. By himself, he is isolated."- Whyte 1880 " A feeling of emptiness comes from our ego's view that we are separate & do not need others, a loss of communication & connectedness develops. This is furthered by TV commercials telling us we are incomplete without their product. JOY is a feeling that is Not connected to outside conditions.." -P. Slater*

Being Positive Takes Energy. When we are Physically 'Depressed', out of energy, It's not possible to be Mentally Positive. Get Physically Strong with Fresh, Quality Food & Sleep so You can be Mentally Positive !

DEPRESSION: A PLACE ? Drug companies have made the term depression into 'a place', the person has 'fallen' into a hole & needs help to get out with Drugs or Therapist. Depression is not a 'place', our energy system gets tired or 'depressed' as our energy 'falls' every few hours, every day; Snack Often, Rest Often..

NEVER ALONE with our 2-sided brain which is 2 personalities, one creative & one analytical. The left side can talk to the right side, the right side cannot talk back, but it can move the left hand. Talking out-loud to oneself is laughed at but it is a helpful process allowing the non-verbal side of our brain to hear our thoughts out-loud & see if they make sense or have wrong thinking, ask yourself if there are other options ? It does not matter if another person is listening, your other brain is ! Write some thoughts down so you can look at them on paper to see if what you are thinking sounds right to yourself. Talk to your other brain, you will never be lonely.

SUICIDAL THOUGHTS ? STOP & Try these first;

- Eat some Ice Cream & Cake & Sit Down & Relax, turn on a comedy on youtube (Jim Gaffigan is very relaxing)

- open a window & get some fresh air and sunshine, do whatever else makes you happy that minute, wash your face.

- notice nature, even on tv, hey, those mountains & clouds are cool, my problems are very small compared to them

- ask yourself out loud: " What else will make me happy now? " answer yourself outloud

- Eat a lot of your favorite foods until you fall asleep

- I suggest a sex session for anyone contemplating suicide. WAIT! then every horny person would say they are suicidal !

Imagine life is like at day at an amusement park. If halfway through we are stung by a bee or get bored, there is still a half-day of fun rides left. Suicide brings nothingness so then enjoying any ride is more fun so let's lower our expectations because anything is more entertaining than nothingness.

" the schizophrenic is drowning in the same waters the mystic swims in with delight " -J. Campbell

REAL MENTAL ANGUISH (vs fake Drama): If we are physically well but are mentally overwhelmed then:

1 Acknowledge we are overwhelmed

2 Understand what is overwhelming us

3 Solve or Rectify the problem, this will take work & time

4 Forgive the situation, do not dwell on it & let it fade

5 Lessons Not Forgotten: Remember where things went wrong so we can avoid that bad direction again.

Positive Statements Vs Complaining Or Moaning; Insecurities hold us back from getting past obstacles: Feel Like Quitting ? Rest & Try Again, negativity holds us back. Realize / Understand that life will always have obstacles & so why waste energy complaining vs focus on getting past the obstacle to our happiness. Maybe we will learn something from the obstacle that will save us time on future obstacles, so calm down & get over it, Work Through the Obstacles.

" Good character is not formed in a short time.
It is created little by little, day by day.
Effort is needed to develop good character " -Heraclitus

Too Much Indoors: For millions of years our brain & eyes neurophysiological development / evolution only experienced rounded forms in nature. There are very few right angles or straight lines in nature. Human buildings have straight lines & rooms are square so our eyes' rods & cones are constantly 'boxed-in' by the the right lines. Subconsciously, our neuropsychology, when we are in buildings, is never fully relaxed. Many conscious architects make buildings with rounded edges & corners; it's easier on our eyes & brains. Get out of 'boxes' & see Nature !

Most Suicides occur in Countries with little SUNLIGHT

Cures for Depression: SUNLIGHT & SLEEP,
a rested & fueled brain can think more clearly and have the energy to face life positively.

SUN POWER: Living things need Sun Light. Skin Infections are healed by sunlight. Modern people spend too much time indoors and have lost their billion year connection to the Power & Necessity of the Sun, it gives us energy & 'vitamins'. Some people have become so mole-like the sun bothers them; expose yourself gradually but get back to being a normal Sun-Loving Animal. All ancient world cultures knew the power of the Sun & worshipped it.

Nature Helps Our Mental Health: One of the many reasons city people get depressed is they have lost a connection with nature, where we lived for millions of years. There is a reason it's called 'Mother' Nature; it is where we came from! Trees, parks, mountains, beaches, rivers; Nature makes us feel nourished, in sync with the rhythm of Life, we feel whole again & it may be the only fresh air / oxygen we get vs office air. read OXYGEN in Osteoporosis section

The vastness of Nature remind us how small we are on this big earth & that our problems are very small compared to the big world. The Benefits of visiting Nature, Physical & Mental are under appreciated: weekly parks visits are better than no nature exposure at all but forests, oceans & jungles should be experienced. *Wilderness* means ' Will of the Place ', will of nature.

NUDE is NATURAL: *" There is a boldness & daring to nudity, a defiant denial of shame. It taps into the sensual power of the body. By reveling in the physical, the ancients reached toward the spiritual. The exhilaration of nudity lifted the ancients closer to the divine. " - D. Angsten*

We Need To Remember That We Are WONDERFUL yet WORTHLESS At The Same Time

Ancient Origin of Negativity: Our earliest experience with nature (night = bad, day = good) led to a misunderstanding of how life has negative in it & that therefore we have negative inside of us which lead to the original sin mythology. Rain floods villages but plants grow, the flood is only negative for some, it's part of life !

NEUROLOGICAL VIEW OF NEGATIVITY: Pathways in the Brain are like paths through a field; they can become deep ruts or overgrown from lack of use. Negative thoughts can recur merely from a negative thought pattern EVEN if that brain pathway is not correct for the new situation! We must catch ourselves from rote actions & feelings & analyze each situation anew. We can create new, positive neural pathways by practicing behavior we want. Depressed people have been found to be stuck in a self-analyzing pattern crowding out the bigger reality of life. Psychedelics open new neural pathways & can break the depressive's negative neural loop to allow a view beyond themselves.

"Meaning of life is being with friends to think & talk together."-Bloom

" Is Life Meaningless? Friendship, Love & Helping Others is Not Meaningless " -Hitchens

Are Animals Lives Meaningless ? Try Taking it Away From Them !

Work Ethics: If our work is causing societal problems that can wear on our soul's sense of justice. Try to find positive work, You're either part of the problem or part of the solution. PS No sunlight or fresh air in offices, get outside for your breaks & Breathe !

TV Consumerism & Materialism Leading to UnHappiness: " *Advertising is ever-increasingly monopolizing our attention, absorbing our capacity for intellectual & emotional reaction, of shaping the habits & imagery of our thoughts, to get us to buy ! Advertising is dominating culture & recreation, the independence of the Press & literary publishing. We are in danger of becoming sluggish intellectually, underdeveloped emotionally, dull & uninteresting to others & ourselves, restless & dissatisfied, incapable of taping into our full strength...Rather than develop us as literature should, advertising warps content, it's purpose is to divert our attention from life's important issues leading to passivity, spectatoritis, undermining active recreation & even warping children's education. " -P. Slater*

" K. Marx saw this: Ownership Superseded Appreciation. We need to move beyond possession, profit & consumerism to have a true experience with people & things, to have a human sensibility, a musical ear, an eye for beauty. " -C. Purnell

1900's: 1st stores with lighted window displays marks mass market beginning of "..purchases Not for necessity but for visual fascination...Modern life became an accumulation of spectacles and social life became about appearances and a superficial existence where people do not connect with real life, a sense of 'having' replaces true interaction. " -R. Bowlby

We Have Over-Developed Brains, We Think Too Much: Over a million years our brains grew/evolved bigger & bigger. Human brains have grown so big they cannot get out of a woman's cervix fully formed so babies are born premature just so that the big head can get out ! Our large, modern brains make our behavior more influenced by our culture & social conditioning. Modern life is so busy with stimulus it is very hard to focus on mind relaxation. Things appear bigger with more thought about them so quiet the brain so it is not whirling in numerous thoughts. Deep breathe & quiet the brain....

EMPOWERING: I've made mistakes & I will make mistakes again but I'm not a quitter so I WILL TRY not to make more mistakes. I'm not perfect but I deserve love because I am trying to do better so I love myself !

" Our dominant paternalistic culture has made us ill with narcissism. Human history has been a 15,000 year dash from the equilibrium of the African cradle to the 20th century apotheosis of delusion, devaluation and mass death. Immersed in junk food, trash media, & cryptofascist politics, condemned to live toxic lives of low awareness. Sedated by TV, they are the living dead, lost to all but the act of consuming, their authenticity lies in obeying mass style changes conveyed through media. We are a part of Nature & Nature is paradise & not to be raped but cherished " " Ideologies are environments of the mind, surrounding & determining for us what we should or can think. " -T. McKenna ' Food of the Gods '

" the grim monotony of american facial expressions-hard, surly & bitter-with an aura of deprivation..weighted down by possessions but acting as if every object they do not own is food they need, the fanatical acquisitiveness.." -P. Slater

Faking anguish to get attention or love ? Maybe some suicidal people are 'spoiled' people who have had it good, got 'spoiled' & then cannot handle any disappointment ? Long process to bring a spoiled person back to the reality that they are no more special than the rest of us & should be happy, or at least content participating in this great adventure, LIFE ! Takes time & work but it can be worked through.

'Serenity is Not freedom from the storm but peace within the storm' -Hopis

" We need to defend against an unfavorable environment, protect the quietness & privacy of our inner world, give ourselves a chance for creativity & self-fulfillment & retain community without which even the strongest person finds it difficult to develop or express theirselves." -G. Keenan 1955

CHILDREN's BRAIN DEVELOPMENT IDEAS

KEEP KIDS OFF ELECTRONIC SCREENS !
The screens scramble the brain's development.

The Brain's Neurons are all there at birth but they diminish if they are not stimulated. The number of neural connections increases with stimulation. Imagine the brain's neural connectors are roots growing from the neurons. The more you stimulate the brain the more extensive & stronger the roots grow, the more neural pathways form, causing a Bigger, More Complex Brain !

Neural Pathways Grow from:

1) **Math & Alphabet Flash Cards** (as early as ? 4 yrs ?) Every child should know by heart ALL Multiplication / Division Tables.

2) **Sports:** Most CAR ACCIDENTS are caused by poor reflexes & poor peripheral vision; GET KID'S COORDINATION TRAINED EARLY with SPORTS ! (kicking a ball is easiest for the youngest. Parents, do it with them, not with coaches until they are advanced. Team Sports Vs Individual Competition: Teams develop cooperation to help each other grow. Individual competition can build character or monsters. Children may not be emotionally ready for the individual pressures.

3) **Music:** banging on a pot lid, piano or drum increases hand-eye coordination & the brain follows the notes, ordering the mind. Do not embarrass your children: NO clarinets, violins, or tubas, ' Use an accordion, go to Jail ! ' -recording studio sign

4) **Foreign Languages:** spanish & french are latin based like english but maybe learn chinese or japanese since they are a whole different system for the brain to learn.

5) **Travel:** Even a walk around the block is better than nothing. Travel book's pictures expand the mind. Books, not screens.

6) **RIGHT BRAIN Exercise:** One side of our brain is non-verbal & underused. Our educational system does not acknowledge the non-verbal brain. We evolved from a right-brain dominant species to a left-brain dominant culture. Modern life's alienation & lack of humane empathy is a symptom of this change. Using the left hand activates the Right Brain Hemisphere. Music is a Right Brain Function. More later.

7) **JUGGLING:** More than hand-eye coordination, juggling is stimulating the brain's 2 sides to do 2 different things, Great !

Learning is Important but it is Important that Learning be Fun !

EDUCATION Should Be: *" A teacher's aim is to make the pupil's mind habits sane, healthy & their whole outlook upon life that of being conscious of their efficiency & being eager & able to solve problems as they arise. The educated person knows more than the average person & is constantly increasing their knowledge while being wary of people with a personal agenda in their ideas. Modern education leads to accepting authority vs Independent thinking.*

Education's goal:

- *learning to SEE & THINK without pre-conceived ideas*

- *learning to DANCE, with feet & WITH WORDS " -Nietzsche*

<u>BREAST FEEDING PREVENTS AIDS, HIV & CANCER</u>

There is no other food with the genetic composition of
HUMAN BREAST MILK !
Mothers have been improving it for Millions of Years !

**Humans & All Mammals receive the fundamental building
blocks of the Immune System through Breast Milk.**
Those Living Human Organisms are Not found in soy or cow's milk,
without them Our Immune System is Deficient.
See HIV & AIDS Section.

Phosphorus: Very Important for Our Big Human Brains & best
found in HUMAN BREAST MILK. Ignore the Fake-Paid-For reports
from Cow & Meat Companies.

A DROP OF BREAST MILK IS BETTER THAN NONE: If you can
only get your baby to taste drops of a human mother's milk the
antibodies enter the child & can replicate. Yes it can be very hard &
painful but keep trying, whatever you have to do to get those
immune system building blocks into the child.

ANY MOTHER's BREAST MILK BETTER THAN NONE:
Throughout human history, any lactating woman in the vicinity
would nurse any hungry child, it broadens the baby's antibody
content & immune system. If need be, another animal's milk is
better than nothing; cow's are dumb, goats are smarter ! In primitive
cultures children would nurse quite late compared to modern terms
without any emotional dependency issues & normal socialization
skills noted.

MILK WAS ONCE BLOOD:
-The food we eat turns into our blood.
-Pregnant Humans & mammals blood turns into their breast milk.
-Drink the blood of Christ -from the christian mass.
-Drinking mother's milk is ingesting their blood, their DNA.
-Ancient people's drank the blood of enemies & sacrificial victims &
strong animals whose power they wanted to ingest, to become a
part of themselves, part of their DNA.

LIVING LIFE THROUGH YOUR CHILD; WHO IS IN CHARGE ?

Parents Should Be a Role Model for the Children, the child is Not the center of the family.

Parents subordinate their own lives to drive children to activities that mostly the parents should be doing WITH their kids. This sends the child a distorted message regarding the value of the kid's activities versus the Parent's worth.

People who have no lives of their own may benefit from being the kid's driver; it gives a purpose to the parents' lives. But it's better to get Adult Hobbies; then your child will have something to be proud of about you versus being the child's servant.

Living Your Life Through Your Child's Life is connected to the idea of a child completing a parent's life. If a parent is lonely, then a child is a blessing, however this is not a normal relationship so be careful to establish boundaries & consult with outside people.

TIME FOCUSED ON THE CHILD's WORLD: Yes, people learn some things from raising a child (enjoy the little things in life, patience), but keep this in mind: every hour you spend in a child's world is an hour you are not moving forward with your own adult life. If the parent is emotionally undeveloped then this dynamic is good for the parent but be aware: raising children slows down the growth of the parent compared to unencumbered adults.

Being with children forces you to be in the moment, their moment. For people whose lives are scattered, children are a very grounding force. Children give purpose to Parents whose lives that have not found purpose yet. Unstable parents may think children are a 'god send'. But that is a BAD reason to have children, therapy is easier.

Genetically, evolutionarily, women are programmed to care for their children. This feeling can extend to other babies & may extend to a desire to nurture any living thing. Nurturing is a wonderful, loving action but my warning is that when there is Only thoughts of nurturing others there is a lack of self-awareness or self-development of one's personality. For some women, they may be content being a care-taker, similar to worker bees whose entire existence is to serve the queen. The emotional reward of attention may be their goal but many may receive their own internal reward as they congratulate themselves for giving. That is Not a fulfilled individual life so be aware. Learning to Love Oneself is what is needed, that takes time,

COLLEGE EDUCATION NOT NECESSARY: Engineers need higher education, but not everyone does. In today's over-populated job market it is important to enter that market as soon as possible to put in the years of hands-on training & experience needed to move forward, Not book learning whose information goes out-of-date by next year vs On-The-Job Intern training which adapts daily to the marketplace. The current fad of demanding college for all is a misguided idea. Young teens, & everyone, need to be trained in a physical skill, or intellectually-minded teens could intern in office or educational settings but everyone still needs to learn a skill with their hands, even accounting but a physical skill is more important to learn; carpentry ? College education is overrated as college years are mostly spent goofing off.

(also see Parenting and Kid's Discipline section)

<u>5G, Cell Towers, WI-FI: Immunity & Brain Damage</u>

Yes, phone radiation is small*, but it's everywhere & constantly increasing, but of course, radiation affects our metabolism & therefore our Immune System, more importantly, Our Brains !

CNN: Earbuds, wireless, found to cause Brain Damage.

-Cell phone use in the car is like having your head inside a microwave oven.

-Never sleep with cell phone switched on beside you, Never even bring the cell phone into the bedroom.

-Using Your Cell Phone a Half Hour Per Day Increases Your Risk of Brain Tumor By 40%

-Avoid carrying your cell phone directly on your body.

Even on standby your cell phone communicates at full power with the nearest cell phone tower regularly (typically several times a second) If you do have to keep your cell phone next to your body keep it away from your major organs. Airplane mode is safer.

Studies show that cell phone radiation and electromagnetic (EMF) exposures can interrupt sleep cycles and contribute to ailments like: irritation of allergies, heart palpitations, muscle pain and weakness, and daytime irritability. These exposures can impede the function of the immune system, reduce the production of melatonin and other hormones and have serious long-term adverse consequences.

https://www.electricsense.com/775/how-to-protect-yourself-from-cell-phone-radiation/

* dentists know radiation damage, they leave the room for x-rays.

YOGA & MEDITATION; THEIR MISUNDERSTANDING

**The desire for perfect yoga poses is the OPPOSITE of what these practices are meant to help us achieve;
Relaxing and Enjoying Life.**

Meditation is a fancy word for Deep Breathing.

Yoga is Stretching our Muscles while Relaxing & Breathing, Turning Off the Mind, or Meditating.

People get caught up in analyzing whether they are doing yoga or meditation the 'right way'. Each person has a different body & mind & each body & mind has it's own 'right way', relaxxxxxxxxxx

Your body type may not be comfortable with some poses, the goal is not achieving a difficult pose, the goal is to release stress, not add the stress of feeling like you're not as good as the person next to you. You are what you are now, be proud of yourself now.

Deep Breathing is the foundation of all spiritual practices & Life ! Our brains evolved into over-analyzing machines which sometimes makes us forget to Deep Breathe. OXYGEN is the most important life nutrient; **Inhale Oxygen Into Your Brain & Muscles.**

Deep Breathing can be done anywhere, even at a red light !

A MANTRA is nothing special, it's just a word repetition to keep your brain from thinking of your life's details; la la la...(see Curb...)

SITTING POSITION is nothing special, lying down has better blood circulation, it's just sitting up we can do more; converse, eat, see. Fingers touching pose ? similar effect as hands clasped which closes or completes the body's bio-electrical current, very subtle.

Ballet, Gymnastics, Olympics Perfectionists: Children molded into their parent's desires in outdated activities with no connection to everyday life or carefree fun. Any pursuit where perfection is the main goal is misguided. We can strive for perfection, but to avoid disappointment we need to recognize that MAYBE we can achieve perfection for one moment but that is not to be expected. Enjoy participating even if we come in last place. ps Gymnastics damages joints & warps fun into competition & approval.

No Pain, No Gain? BAD ADVICE ! Overdoing exercise is how most injuries occur. **Pain is how the body communicates with our brain saying " Stop It ! "** The correct exercise goal is to push ourselves a little but Not to the point of pain. Extra exertion, doing one more push-up than normal makes the muscle grow one level stronger during the next day's recovery / rest period, HOWEVER, so many enthusiasts forget their common sense & overdue often causing not only superficial injuries but potentially deep-tissue injuries. Do not follow TV Sport Product Commercials with their ' do it all now ! ' mentality; 50 year old former athletes trying to be young again & damaging their older bodies, see ego pages.

INVERSION / STANDING ON YOUR HEAD: Silly. yes, more blood goes to your head, a head rush, but it is Not natural for our head to receive that much blood. Many better ways to get a 'head rush', like breathing & exercising or dancing ! The muscle control is amazing but it's a show-off trick or silly fad. PS blood goes to your head when you lay down ! put your head over the edge of your bed !

" Meditation is Weird " It's a weird word, it makes it all sound so spiritual & mysterious. Maybe if it was called DEEP BREATHING it would not seem so weird.

BE HERE NOW: We seem to never be thinking of the moment we are experiencing; we think about what we are about to do or say, what we said, the past, but not the air we're breathing. " If your memory holds your reality, then as your memory reduces, your reality reduces. " " ....the idea of destiny is lazy, not taking responsibility..." -C. Klosterman

<u>CHIROPRACTIC DAMAGE / INJURIES BEST TREATMENT</u>

<u>Chiropractic Can Be Damaging VS Massage</u>

Cracking Our Joints Does Make Them Bigger & Then They Are More Likely To Go Out Of Position In The Future.

Hands On Physical Therapy is the best healing methodology: Gently massaging limbs that are out of alignment is better than cracking the joints but massage takes more of the doctor's time & is seen as beneath doctors because anyone can massage. Gentle manipulation (Swedish technique) of the damaged area heals best, stimulating blood into the damaged area. Joint cracking may occur during gentle manipulation, but if a masseuse is too hard or too soft let them know, you are paying. That will lead to a Happy Ending !

ICE INJURIES RIGHT AWAY & ELEVATE for 24-48 hours.

STOPPING THE BLOOD FLOW to the damaged area in the first MINUTES, HOURS & DAYS is the MOST IMPORTANT TIME of the healing. If you focus on slowing blood flow to the damaged and surrounding areas until the torn capillaries 'knit' back together your recovery time will be shorter, sit on the couch for a day & heal faster

Longer Injury Recovery occurs because the blood that oozed out of the torn capillaries is now trapped in the damaged area. The quicker the area is iced after the injury the less blood flows out through the torn capillaries. There are 100's of little blood vessels and pain means some of them have been torn.

BRUISING & SWELLING is the blood that has flowed out of the damaged capillaries staying in the damaged area.

After the capillaries 'knit' back together (heal) the blood that flowed out of the tiny torn blood vessels is TRAPPED there & has to then be removed molecule by molecule through the cell walls, a very slow process. Capillaries knit back together in 36-48 hours. Warm water and epson salts after 2 days to get that trapped blood out.

A SPRAIN / INJURY / BREAK damages;

1) Capillaries
2) Corpuscles
3) Muscle Fibers
4) Tendon Fibers

KEEP Injured Area COLD & ELEVATED 2-3 days to stop more blood from going into the damaged area. NOT TOO COLD so that it is uncomfortable otherwise the body thinks the area is freezing & rushes blood to the cold area, the opposite of what we want.

Alternate Warm & Cold AFTER the capillaries knit back together, (depending on severity, 36-48 hours). Aternating temperature increases flow of blood with it's healing nutrients & cleaning trapped blood out of the area. (but ONLY COLD for at least 1 day)

Shin Splints / Shin Pain / Knee Pain; Landing hard on your Heels causes the impact to go straight up the leg instead of landing on the Ball of the foot absorbing the shock before transferring weight to the heel. Look at the construction of the leg; impact on the heel goes straight up to the shin & knee. Change your running pattern & pain will go away...step 'lightly on the earth'.

BROKEN BONES take a long time to knit back together, molecule by molecule. Do Not push a break too much too early, the break probably happened because we were in a Hurry ! Slow Down & Smell the Flowers.... Fresh nutrients, green veggie juices are the best, fast injection of minerals & vitamins to give the injury nutrients.

EPSON SALTS: Soaking in any kind of salt draws out toxins and / or trapped blood from injuries. Water temperature should be comfortable, not too hot.

Burns: Immediately & for 24-36 hours place burn in cool / cold water, literally allowing the skin to absorb molecule by molecule, the water that was burned away. Immerse burn in cool water as long as possible, in the bathtub if needed. You must have heard that butter feels good.

ULTRASOUND is RADIATION; it is known to break up calcification but at what effect to surrounding cells ? The dosages & side effects need more research, over decades. It's another machine doctors can charge for & the therapists do not have to use their muscles & work to carefully massage the injury, which is the best therapy; Hands On. The hands have electrical energy also, Healing Hands !

TIRED vs LETHARGIC:

TIRED means muscles are out of carbo energy & need to rest & re-fuel.

LETHARGIC means our blood has slowed down & we are 'listless'. Our muscles have energy in them but are not ' in gear', we need to get ourselves moving.

If you are TIRED, rest & eat.

If you are LETHARGIC, MOVE YOUR LAZY ASS ! A Musical 'Beat' Makes Us Want to Move, Put on Your Favorite Dance Music !

PERFECTIONISTS / TOUGH GUYS / ASKING FOR HELP

LAUGHING AT OUR MISTAKES / BEING DIFFERENT

Perfectionists not only make their own lives more difficult, they make life more difficult for those they deal with. Our lives are not going to be perfect & contorting ourselves to try to achieve perfection is unrealistic & a pain for everyone. We can strive towards perfection & maybe achieve it in small areas, but we need to be aware that the perfection we have in mind may be too much trouble to achieve & may keep us from moving on to something else that may be even better for us. Continual striving for perfection takes focus away from enjoying life as it is & as we are.

'Tough Guy' Persona; trapped in one personality; they can never be whimsical or silly or carefree. Constantly guarding their emotions to act 'tough' suppresses parts of themselves & builds tension in them so when they are pressured they Snap ! & take it out on us !

ASKING FOR HELP / RECEIVING HELP: The attitude of "I am self-sufficient & do not need anyone", the John Wayne, James Dean macho-man persona, is widespread. For insecure people it is a persona to hide behind, or a mating strategy to attract women ? A wise person knows they can always learn & that we all are only here from the help of our past families. Also, Sharing is Fun !

BEING DIFFERENT: It is hard to be different in a society where it causes gossip, scorn or jealousy. *" a person gifted with a creative imagination is cast into a solitary freak-like role in society "* -Karlinsky on Nabokov - *" The Charm of an Uncommon Personality in Free Form, Unhindered by Convention "* -Mencken

A Person Must Be Strong To Argue With Society.

CHANGING YOUR MIND is a sign of a brain that has the flexibility, the neurological adaptability to be able to stop & realize a new idea is better and then adjusting; evolution is adjusting / adapting to a new environment. The 'Tough Guy' is socially inhibited from changing their mind for fear of being seen as 'wishy-washy', spineless, weak. They are afraid of what other's think because of a lack of confidence from a lack of self love, probably going back to early years lack of love.

Why don't people want to admit their mistakes ? It opens them up to being ridiculed, they think being made fun of diminishes their worth. Anyone who thinks a person making a mistake is not worthwhile is not worth having as a friend. Business relations more complicated...

Can We Handle being LAUGHED AT ?

Can We Laugh AT OURSELVES?

The Value of the Jester / Trickster: The jester offers himself up for ridicule with the goal that people laughing at the jester can learn to laugh at their own foibles, rather than go negative when mistakes happen. Accepting that we are not perfect, that we all make mistakes, that life has tragedy but we can still laugh at it if we remember the bigger, solar system picture; that we're only alive for a short time. It is important to remember our weaknesses; so our egos do not get too big...Jon ! (see J. Campbell video series)

Humble Attitude:

1 I know I lack knowledge, I can sometimes be stupid, slow, a fool, an idiot.

2 By accepting I am not perfect, instead of beating myself up over my errors, I can find amusement in my errors, so,

3 It does not hurt me if others laugh at my errors also.

4 Love Yourself & You Always Have Love, don't let the turkeys weigh you down.

" Art has the Right to be Pure Foolishness, Pure Foolishness is Therapeutic " -Nietzsche & Wagner

Recovering Perfectionist Mottos:

1) I've made mistakes & I will make mistakes again but I'm not a quitter so I will try not to make more mistakes.

2) I'm not perfect but I still love myself & I deserve love because I am trying to be better.

3) My life is not perfect but I do not criticize myself, I work to improve my life every chance I get. There is an ideal I can strive for but I do Not expect to reach it & I sometimes enjoy 'unhealthy' habits because " Everything in Moderation, Including Moderation ! " was that Sinatra ? " We Got to Cut Loose Sometimes Man ", was that Sammy ?

BEING DOGMATIC: It is easy to be dogmatic when we have some evidence but yet we may not know every opposite view. Exception: Mass killers; No other valid view on their guilt. Similar to the 'Wise Child Complex': acting either bored or preachy.

Roman Humility Tradition: Roman Generals returning victorious from war to the adoring roman crowds had in their chariot a hidden servant repeating: " All Fame Is Fleeting " to keep the generals egos down to earth. Romans always let their conquered tribes worship whatever gods they wanted, but no god exempt from tax, smart.

COMPLAINERS: It gives them a rush of power. There is revenge in complaining. Anarchists blame the gov't. & christians blame their original sin, always something besides their own actions. " *The christian 'last judgement' is the ultimate revenge of the downtrodden* " -Nietzsche

HATE TRANSFER: If you receive hate from a person for no logical reason, it probably comes from their past, your behavior triggers it. It's not logically based, the deeper connections must be sorted through; may take lots of time.

BIG EGOs:

mostly from low self-esteem, desire for attention:

MOUNT EVEREST: Are you a failure if you do not reach the top ? The 2000 people who have died climbing it must have thought so. What a silly, ego driven objective. And all the other death defying actions people take for a 'rush' of excitement ? Is it because their nervous system's are 'maxed out' from caffeine & stimulants & they need to feel higher excitement to feel something special in their lives ? Or Ego desire for attention ? The goal is supposed to be THE VIEW from a high place but all they see is the climber in front of them ! Obvious disregard for their loved ones...

TATTOOS: An obvious cry for attention. The social pressure inside the 'parlor' to 'ink-up' must be strong or the 'parlor's' attention socially addictive, as in needing friends. BAD NEWS: That ink slowly drips into the blood stream, molecule by molecule, poisoning the system & brain. Interesting how many tattooed people frequent health food establishments ? Try a temporary tattoo or clothes with a pattern before committing, you can change clothes !

BALLET, GYMNASTICS, OLYMPICS PERFECTIONISTS: Repeated here: Children molded into their parent's desires in outdated activities with no connection to everyday life or carefree fun. Any pursuit where perfection is the main goal is misguided. We can strive for perfection, but to avoid disappointment we need to recognize that MAYBE we can achieve perfection for one moment but that is not to be expected. Enjoy participating even if we come in last place. ps Gymnastics damages joints & warps fun into competition & approval.

RUN or WALK FAST ? You do Not have to run to exercise, walking fast burns calories too, go at a pace your body is comfortable with, and that can vary day to day based on sleep, carbos, sex, etc.

YOGA perfection & a competitive mindset is the OPPOSITE of what these practices are meant to help us with; to Relax & Enjoy Life. see full yoga section, pg 89.

AGING ATHLETES: A 40 year-old body cannot perform as well as it did at 25 years ! Joint braces or back braces or Pills that sell you on continuing physical movements from your 20's are selling the 'fountain of youth' to you. Your 40 yr old body is not supposed to be running hurdles or doing gymnastics anymore ! Exercise smoothly & you will not have joint injuries. Allow rest days for muscles to replenish, over-working muscles tears them down.

Resting Is Not Weakness, It Is Recharging & Healing.

WOMEN's WORKOUTs or MEN'S: Females should not want to & genetically / biologically are not made to bulk up like a man, women should tone & strengthen without acquiring bulk. Of course genetic testosterone levels vary.

REPETITIVE Movements: BAD. Muscles are not evolved to do the same movement over & over; that never occurs in nature. Keep your movements varied as each muscle is made up of HUNDREDS of strands & each movement variation strengthens different strands.

FINGERNAILS PERFECT ? The obsession over fingernails & toenails is damaging to them. Appreciate your natural nails, nevermind getting compliments from other girls & let your nails breathe ! Excessive make-up clogs pores; let your pores breathe !

WOMEN ACCEPTING COMPLIMENTS: Most women, and some men, have a hard time accepting a compliment. Self-Love or Pride is seen by puritan thought as 'sinful' or Insecure people do not want attention. The usual response to a compliment is self-deprecating; " oh this old dress.." WOMEN: Just respond " Thank You ! " whew, was that so hard ? Other bad habit; Women critiquing themselves so they do not have to bear hearing another person speak of their flaws & embarrassing them. Do Not say anything bad about Yourself, we all have flaws, do not focus on them, Say Positive Things About Yourself ! (see 'The Beauty Myth' N. Klein)

Personality Types:

1) A-HOLES / JERKS: Pushing one's ideas even when one knows other people are upset with their ideas. CONFUSING: You can be correct about a subject & still be an A-Hole / Jerk if you are not respectful of others who have not had the same opportunities to learn as much.

2) SPOILED BRAT: given everything without working for it, willing to push someone out to get ahead, only has compassion for others when it suits them.

3) COMPASSIONATE / CARING; will not go ahead if someone else deserves it. *" when we're really compassionate we do not want to hurt animals either " Einstein*

4) GIVES TOO MUCH / MARTYR: inconveniences themselves to give to another, caused by desire for attention usually from a lack of self-love. What if people suffer but do not want to listen to advice ? should one be forceful (a jerk ?) to get the people to go the right way for their own good ? (example; forcing people away from a road that leads to a sink-hole)

5) " Person whose dominance is higher than their intelligence or imagination so that they feel they deserve high merit but they lack the insight to see that they do not deserve high merit. " - C. Wilson

Feel sorry for these people but their issues affect us all:

- Intellectuals who get trapped in the belief they need to always appear smart to make themselves unique or special or necessary, above or apart from the world. They are unwilling to participate in the simple joy of playing in the sand or a swimming pool because their intellectual identity might be undermined by being seen as frivolous.

- Driving rude ? Most speeding drivers are late for an appt. or listening to speed rock, let them Go ! For people who have no real control of their lives, driving makes them feel powerful & they can act rude. Depart for your destination early so you can drive relaxed & play some nice music to keep you calm. See TEENS CANNOT DRIVE & TALK sec.

Are We Special ? *" one of the oldest & deepest american psyche myths is the fantasy of being special. The unstated aspect of " do your own thing " is that everybody will be watching us; that a special superiority will be acknowledged by others...we need to abandon these narcissistic dreams. " -P. Slater 'Pursuit of Loneliness'*

REMEMBERED in the future? Worry that our life is meaningless, that we will be forgotten after our death, leads people to do silly things; build monuments, act in in illogical ways solely for posterity, even a motivation for having children. Do not act for an unknown future, there is no proof of anything for us beyond our grave.

HAVING CHILDREN for POSTERITY ? We understand the ego wanting immortality through offspring. But consider fish who fertilize the eggs in mid-air, never feel any contact or ever see their offspring; what type of biological drive did that develop from ? ego ?

" Self-Respect comes from the willingness to accept responsibility for one's life (one's actions). The greatest power of Self-Respect is that it frees us from the expectation of others. Self-Respect gives Moral Nerve " -Didion

Earn Self-Respect by being a good person. Self-Love comes from Self-Respect so we do not need to act tough or perfect to try to gain respect from others because we have our own respect already.

Confidence comes from Respecting Ourselves.
We Respect Ourselves when we have Done Good Things.
(but criminals can respect their good crimes...needs education)

Intelligent VS Smart: A Smart person can learn things, can be clever. However there is the difference between learning to fix a problem VS Creating a New Solution. It takes INTELLIGENCE to think of a new solution & then further to think of how to implement the solution to fix the problem. The term 'Intellectual' is often used negatively referring to people stuck in their heads without real-world experience or common sense in dealing with life; that is a **PHILOSOPHER.** An INTELLECTUAL is someone who devises, creates & offers solutions to life's & societies' problems. Example; George Orwell, great thinker who went to war for his beliefs.

" PHILOSPHY comes from those who are thinking too much, they are Not acting in society, they are only thinkers & their thoughts reflect their in-active, incomplete lives." -Nietzsche

*" God is a comedian playing to an audience who will not laugh "
-Voltaire (funny because Voltaire was an atheist !)*

ALCOHOLISM & DRUG ADDICTION: NO EXCUSES !

A 'Buzz' is Fun ! Discipline Is What Stops Us From Hurting Ourselves.

The BUZZ from Alcohol, 'Upper' Drugs & Sugar are from the same neural receptors. All living organisms respond to sugar, it is an energy booster, it makes life more active, we do more, but there is the 'come-down', when we rest & eat & get ready to go again.

The only thing stopping us from over-consuming is mental discipline. The Mind CAN tell the hand muscles to STOP ingesting the bad stuff ! Just because junk is in front of you, it does Not mean you have to consume it, DISCIPLINE !

A Brain cannot think clearly & have Discipline if it does not have the nutrients to function properly. The Nutrient that our brains have run on for 13,000 years is the B-Complex found in Whole Grains. Meat companies have paid congress & the FDA & paid for ads to distort the info on the B-Complex. The Brain needs the B-Complex from Whole Grains, NOT processed, pulverized whole grain bread or pasta.

Mental Discipline, Correct Thinking, Comes From A Properly Nourished Mind / Brain !

If a person is properly nourished they are less inclined to desire an energy boost, they already have energy, they feel fine. Feed 'addicts' healthy food & watch their discipline grow day by day !

ADDICTS ? I do not like to use the term ADDICTS because this implies the person is powerless. Each use of the drug is a decision. It is LACK of DISCIPLINE which leads to drug use; Drugs don't kill people, people kill themselves with drugs. Every person has a different genetic & psychological history so your parents' habits need to be understood to understand your own.

COFFEE, SUGAR, TOBACCO; Many addicted to these have quit, the same discipline used on these will work on stronger drugs also.

ALCOHOL can be fun or used to aid sleep but it's a POISON so keep it to a minimum. Distilled spirits kill & will cause vision problems; Blind Drunk ! Wine & beer are more natural. Alcohol has been loved since before writing existed for it's psychologically freeing effects, as you know ! CNN VIDEO FOOTAGE: Animals eat fermented fruit, get a buzz & are seen staggering to their sleep.

" 1st alcohol drink makes you Fun !

2nd drink makes you Wild !

3rd drink makes you lose control & act like an idiot

4th drink, You Are a Fool " - GQ

'Alcoholic' generally refers to a person unable to control their life. However athletes & intellectuals drink a lot, to disengage from the physical tension in muscles & mental tension in brains. I think a clarified term for ALCOHOLIC is needed. A 'Functioning Alcoholic' is different from a homeless wino. Tea-totalers hate alcohol drinker's over-the-top behavior so they call them alcoholics even though it is the behavior that they dislike. Drinkers think tea-totalers are boring prudes.

" I decided to drink alcohol because it stopped me from being bored – it stopped other people from being boring to me. Alcohol would make me want to prolong the conversation and enhance the moment...." -C. Hitchens

VISION PROBLEMS will come from Excessive Alcohol, Sugar, Toxins. Blood flows through the eye's veins carrying good nutrients but also toxins which 'cloud' the eye's lens, so eat less sugar & junk food, see ? ps The Eye has muscles for focusing; when we wear glasses to do the focusing the eye muscles get weaker; wear glasses as little as possible.

<u>SEX ADDICTION / LOVE ADDICTION: NO EXCUSES 2 !</u>

We All Should Enjoy Love & Physical Contact, Sexual &/or Massages.

Discipline Is What Stops Us From Excess.

Sex Addiction: Having sex to feel psychologically loved is a problem. 1st step: learn to love yourself by being a good person worthy of Love. If You do Not Love Yourself, Why Should Anyone Else Love You ? Read next 3 pages & other Psychology sections.

Sex Need has Increased in the 50 Years that Steroids & Hormones have been put in meat, milk, eggs & cheese causing high testosterone levels & excessive sex desires. Extra Protein intake also a factor. Steroids causes increased physical need VS this section being about the mental aspect of desiring excessive sex.

Love Addiction: never being loved & then craving love or attention ? that's not an Addiction ! That is from bad upbringing that can be healed through learning to love yourself. When we love ourselves we do not depend on another's love. However, the love from others is always nice to have IN ADDITION to loving yourself.

Love From Others Will Come As You Do Good Things, Selfish People Do Not Deserve Love !

Sex Education: All of us need to have a healthy view of sex within the contexts of love, respect & self-love. The religious view that loving sex is bad must be changed, see Religion section. Teach children that sex is natural & a normal, healthy part of our lives. Love of Self is the basis of healthy living, being a healthy person. If you have old, outdated views of sex then you should get help teaching your child.

Sex created life before religion existed. Ignore stupid religious threats of their made-up HELL or their attempts to control our sex lives which can be life-scarring to young children & adults. Religion gives people hope but their dogmatism is horrible: " Our God, Not Yours ! " Masturbation is how a person learns about their body through practicing & preparing to touch another person lovingly. The practice of buying a 16yr old boy a prostitute is better than no advice or instruction.

Excessive Focus On The Genitalia: Full Orgasms are Whole-Body Orgasms, experiencing stimulating sensations of all the cells in our bodies. Usually, like sports or music, physical awareness & control takes time & practice. Interesting: A man can experience a full-body orgasm with zero fluid release; this is a body-centric sensation VS genital.

CONTROLLING SEX: We learn to regulate our orgasms through practice, especially masturbation, learning to postpone ejaculation & even delaying it by a few days depending on your energy level.

VASECTOMY: Blocking body passages will cause long-term damage from side-effects. Youngsters should learn sexual control through masturbation. Complicated subject, read on.

Oral Sex: This is an important subject in a person's psychological development because a person cannot be fully free unless they are fully physically free / open. There are psychological, societal &/or emotional reasons a person might be uncomfortable with oral sex, however, evolutionarily it is a natural part of our sex lives.

Anal Sex: All body parts should enjoy touching but I think the anus should not be stretched, any permanent stretching can only cause changes / problems in the future, especially as people grow older, similar to cracking knuckles making them bigger. Touching should be pleasant. A desire for excessive pain is not healthy, talk it out.

America's Puritanical Problem, Religious Moralizing: 3/4ths of the world has multiple wives & state sanctioned mistresses; the religious moralizing in america has warped the whole societies' morals & values. Let's continue to work to un-do their negative influence.

" ..from the crucifixion of christ, the prophet of Total Love, it took 300 years to the transformation of his message into a political power (Catholic Church) that kills Love of the Body, until the Renaissance starts loving the body again..." ..the sexual orgasm is the key to psychological health...(Jon's note: a virgin has not experienced full life so can not be full mentally, emotionally or obviously physically....but not all neuroses come from sex issues)

" Self-Consciousness, embarrassment of our naked, natural bodies, is the fall from Grace, (the story of) expulsion from the garden of eden where we lived without embarrassment.. " -W. Reich

ROMANCE LOST: " In the relations between the sexes all beauty is founded on romance, all romance founded upon mystery, and all mystery founded upon ignorance or, upon the deliberate denial of the known truth.To be in love is to be in a state of perpetual anesthesia. " " Make the young suffer the Monotony of Monogamy, that will dampen their passions " -H.L. Mencken

Orgy Described: *" My body ignited in a blaze of sensation. Thought was entirely obliterated. It seemed I could no longer see-only hear, smell, taste, touch. Everything blurred....I lost all sense of separation, of being bound in a single sheath of skin. " - D. Angsten & description of Love as " mindless misery, infantilizing & delusive "*

Goddess Culture Studies point out that our sexual dysfunctions start from our *" ..social system that teaches men and women to equate true masculinity with dominance and violence. " -R. Eisler ' Chalice and the Blade '.*

SICK ? FOR ATTENTION ?

For real physical sickness, look in the Table of Contents for your health issue but this section is about the psychology of someone labeling themselves a sick person to get attention instead of changing themselves into a person worthy of attention.

Getting Attention Through Acting Sick: Maybe being sick got someone attention & maybe that attention was received as Love. A craving for external love stays in people UNTIL THEY LEARN TO LOVE THEMSELVES & don't have to crave it from others. If you are that type of person that enjoys the attention of being sick, be aware that after you get the attention everyone wants to be away from you. Pity makes the recipient wallow in their negative situation instead of encouraging them to face the difficulty & figure out a solution. Perhaps the person missed childhood approval, affection. Whatever it was: Move Forward to Loving Yourself ! " I have faults but I will try to be better and I love and respect myself for working to be better ."

" I'm Going to Beat that Cancer or other disease ! " Your immune system became weak & bacteria / viruses are taking over. Strengthen your immune system 'fighters' with fresh food's vitamins & minerals (not vitamin pill's dead dust), then your 'fighters' will destroy the ' out of control ' bacteria / viruses. Blood Flow, Circulation to body problems will clean out & heal. Make Your Blood Watery, Not fatty, greasy blood, so it Flows to the problem areas. Fresh Vegetable Juices Heal Fastest, pay Whole Foods Juicer $5/day for 2 Weeks, buy it fresh, only bottled if no fresh available.

PARENTS / HEREDITARY BAD EATING: (repeated here) People may say about a sick person: " His father had that disease, the son got it or caught it too ". If the father ate fatty sausage every day & the child grew up eating fatty sausage, when they both have heart attacks people say: " they have a family history of heart disease " when they should say " they have a family history of eating Fatty Foods ! " Bad Health can be changed, even if someone is born with bad organs, by not repeating the bad habits of the ancestors.

<u>Lying or Making Things Up & NOT Knowing It !</u>

<u>Split-Brain Experiments:</u>

The Corpus Callosum is a bundle of nerves that connect the Left Brain & the Right Brain. 1960's seizure victims had their Corpus Callosums cut to stop their seizures & then were given social experiments with their consent. Cutting the CC stops the 2 brain sides from communicating with each other. The Brain's Right Side is verbal; controlling the mouth & spatial relations. The Brain's Left Side is analytical & does Not control the mouth but controls the right side of the body.

Experiment Steps Performed on 30 Subjects with similar results:

1) Brain's verbal left hemisphere controls the right eye & with left-eye covered, the right eye was shown picture of red apple
2) non-verbal hemisphere right brain controls left eye & it was shown picture of yellow car with right-eye covered.

Researcher: what did you see ?
Subject responds verbally, the right eye saw: " apple "
Researcher: draw what you saw with your left hand, the non-verbal
Subject with LEFT-HAND then draws a car
Researcher: why did you draw car when you said you saw apple ?
Subject: because my 1st car was apple red (Not the Reason !)

CONCLUSION: The Subject made up a LIE to justify what HIS OWN hand drew ! This Proves People will make things up to explain their actions. People have been found to lie and not be aware they are lying, their mind's wiring is mis-firing, they are deluding themselves, scary.

MORE LIES: The left brain is always searching for a pattern or reason for what is happening & it will invent a rationale to explain random events & may INVENT DETAILS that were not there, usually from the memory of a similar past situation. This is what organized religion does to explain the randomness of earthquakes killing people: religions says people were bad so god killed them.

<u>HAPPY ? YOU BETTER BE !</u>

Happiness Is The Feeling Of Contentment We Have Because We Are Glad That We Are Alive !

If Someone is Not Happy to be Alive, they have never faced Death.

If Your Life is not under threat,
there is No Excuse for you to be anything but HAPPY !

Happiness is often confused with exaltation or being ecstatic; which we all should feel at special times in our lives, maybe even at some point every day. Ecstasy is an escape from the mental repetition of our daily life. Music can be one of our Ecstasies. Enjoying nature's wonders can be another ecstasy. But that is not what is meant by Happiness, which is a general, sustained, contented feeling. Happy is Not ecstatic, it is contented, Happy.

Physical & Psychological are intertwined so to be fully, deeply Happy we need a properly functioning body & a mind with a contented understanding of our small place in this vast universe. It is hard to feel happy when we are constantly chasing goals our ego has been conditioned by a narcissistic society & TV ads to want fame, wealth, big house, etc.

Q: Can we be really Happy if we are physically sick ?

A: NO. a person can project happiness but that is a facade if their physical sickness is 'eating away' at them psychologically & emotionally. Maybe they try to forget but until they are well with the correct internal balance of protein, carbos, vitamins, cholesterol, salt, etc. they will be off-balance, Physically & Psychologically. If a sick person is working towards recovery then they can be happy about that progress but keep working.

Q: Can we still be Happy if we are under stress ?

A: Yes we can be happy under stress; lack of rent can put us on the streets but we are happy to be alive & not in a war zone, so we should remain fundamentally happy.

Q: Why do people say they are Not Happy?

A: These people have lost connection with life, they have stopped noticing the wonder of life; trees, clouds. Their minds have become conditioned by fantasy thoughts (from TV?) & they are no longer thrilled with the wonder of being alive; we call them whining complainers or losers. These people need hard work to earn their food & remember their small place in this big life. A Sense of Entitlement causes those to feel they 'deserve' better & then when they do not receive their 'fantasy' they become bitter & depressed & take it out on others, who they may feel are 'in their way'.

In modern society happiness is seen as a private, personal term. Sociologists write of primitive villages where an individual's bad luck affects the village. If a whole village is sad can an individual in that village be happy ? We think of ourselves too much & not of our place in our community, if we ever get a chance to have a community.

Life is better with a positive attitude,

you can fight the river's current or enjoy the ride.

" overcome self-division, become undivided & harmonious."-Wilson

Ethics, Bad Behavior & Happiness: What If we know what we are doing with our life is wrong ethically; causing others pain to benefit ourselves. (tobacco emplyee, etc) A person may be ok but on a sub-conscious level, deep down in their core, that deceit will cause them internal dis-ease. Outmaneuvering an opponent is different than lying to win. I propose the liar will have an internal negative affecting them. But what if the person lying thinks that lying in business is fair & does not feel bad, will the negative action still be working within his subconscious ??

WHAT IS THE MEANING OF LIFE ? What is the meaning of Blue ? Why are we here ? Our logical brains ask these questions but the universe is too big for us to comprehend so we have to let these questions go. We place meaning on the universe because our thoughts have meaning for us, but the Sun is Not thinking of Meaning. Our Lives Do Not Matter to a Tree.

People that rely on religious stories for lifes meaning should relax by understanding that their lives are not being judged by a man in the sky. Religious people try to explain " It's God's Will for Babies to be Killed in War ". That is a crazy answer to justify their god beliefs. There is no meaning to the killing of babies in war, it's random, just like life. Most people would rather argue than think through their beliefs rationally. Be nice, try your best & leave the place better than when you arrived. Let's Quit Over-Thinking Life & Enjoy it ! La Vida Es Corta, DisFruitarla!

Animal Happiness: Silly naturalists ask why animals play around, why they jump, why dolphins surf !! They are having Fun !

" MEANING OF LIFE: Being with friends & to think & talk together "
-Bloom

<u>**PARTY DRUGS, PSYCHEDELICS; Positive & Negative**</u>

Illegal drugs may not be purchased or consumed.

LSD, Ecstasy, MDNA: lab-made, often have additives that cause Brain Damage (horse tranquilizer, strychnine)

**" Psychedelics help with Mental Problems, Depression "
-NYU & JOHN HOPKINS Universities**

Psychedelic Mushrooms / Peyote / Psilocybin / Marijuana: All these have grown in nature for millions of years and have been used globally shown by 20,000 year old cave paintings of mushrooms.

The Goal of Psychedelics: Our large logical brains see our bodies as separate from nature, the world & other people. Psychedelics open our senses so that we realize that plants are breathing also & we are not the center of life & the best course of action is to Enjoy That We Are Alive ! The energy rush from the psychedelics can override our day-to-day societal inhibitions, like alcohol. With this bigger perspective it can help people face the bigger, cosmic picture including illnesses, personality issues & taboos like death.

" Psychedelics main benefits are; (D. Pinchbeck)

- our neural receptors / senses open wider & we see that plants breathe & animals think like us, giving us greater levels of empathy to all of life
- a wider intellectual scope (brain areas talk to each other, so we see broader connections) bringing visionary insights
- a more refined aesthetic & sensuous engagement with the physical world
- dissolution of ego boundaries, hopefully longterm
- deconditioning from proscribed social roles " (realizing we do not need to follow others & can choose for ourselves)

2 Personalities Helped by Psychedelics Therapy:

1) Egoist / Bad Social Behavior: The effect of opening their cells lets in the big outside and they see / feel that they are Not the center of the Universe. The Egotistical become more humane, more empathetic towards others.

2) Introvert: Seeing their own energy shows them they are as worthwhile a part of the universe as the next person, they are empowered.

The above lessons can be learned without psychedelics but a lifetime of negative conditioning coded into neural pathways can make change hard. Psychedelic substances re-activate Neural pathways that have 'crusted over' from lack of use or neural pathways that were never engaged because of societal blocks on dance or music or smelling life ! Besides neural blocks there are linguistic blocks to experiencing life in full. Some cultures do not even have the term ' I '. For them, there is no individual, we're all part of the world.

From prolonged, focused thinking we may be able to see negative patterns that should be changed & see new, better patterns of behavior. This is not magic or the drugs, this is the positive result of thinking. Speaking out-loud makes ideas clearer even if we are saying them out-loud from one brain hemisphere to another, called ' Talking to Oneself ', useful.

A Balanced, Healthy Person does not need drugs to be content, they are calm, contented, happy from oxygen into their brains & flower's smells & colors are a bonus. Fundamentally this book is trying to steer us all there. Anyone can achieve calm through relaxing & breathing fresh air but most people are too impatient to relax, calm down & take a breather. Lot of songs about Breathing...

MARIJUANA: 50% of USA & many countries recognize the medical benefits the Chinese have documented for 5,000 Years (Malaria, Rheumatism, INSOMNIA). The 'high' or 'buzz' is the flooding of our system with our stored glycogen energy released by the THC. The extra glycogen sugar opens all our receptor cells, pores, brain, which allows us to see, feel & hear more vibrations than usual; that is the psychedelic experience. The amount of glycogen energy we have stored will determine how long 'the high' lasts and then comes drowsiness & sleep. If we are 'run down', drugs will produce little 'buzz' because we have no stored glycogen to release.

Marijuana is the Antidote to Excess Testosterone.

Fun fact: 8,000 BC mummy found in China with 5 ft marijuana plant in his coffin ! (sad: wife & servants buried alongside)

ART, CREATIVITY & PSYCHEDELICS: Drugs release our stored energy, our stored complex sugar glycogen, which opens all our cells wider. Animals senses are open wider than humans so they hear & smell more vibrations. Our cells opened wider allow us to receive more vibrations, like a stronger radio receiver. Open cells feel textures deeper / smell odors deeper / experience more of the worlds vibrations.

Also, New neural pathways are opened that cause interaction of brain areas not normally communicating with each other. This causes the 'creative insights' users refer to. Smell memory neurons & sight memory neurons 'talk' to each other for the 1st time. Famous psychedelic quote " I Smell Yellow ". Yellow is a specific vibration. This same experience has been verified among a unique group of non-drugged people, they see green when they hear a certain sound, without drugs ! This brain condition is called synesthesia showing that brain wiring is flexible, the neurons are like soft plastic, thus the term Neural-Plasticity, my favorite study subject at UC & the fundamental idea of this book; That we Can Change Ourselves, little by little, Our Neurons are Malleable !

? BAD TRIP ? You Can Stop Negative Thoughts from Circulating In Your Brain by Overriding them with Positive Thoughts. A drug, even sugar, can cause deep-rooted, unresolved negative issues to come forward. If this happens just continually repeat positive ideas & try to find & work through their negative source. see Depression sec.

" the schizophrenic is drowning in the same waters the mystic swims in with delight " - J. Campbell.

HALLUCINATIONS: (from drugs, sleep deprivation, fasting, chanting, drumming, ayahuasca, alcohol) are seen as magical But they are Not. They are just projections from our mind, from our past, our memories, things we heard &/or imagined, nothing more than apparitions of the mind.

SHAMANS: Sensitive or Experienced or Educated People who help the majority of people who are not as fully aware of life's issues.

ALTERNATE REALMS ? OTHER REALITIES ? Wise or educated men & women were trying to say, for example, that a plant may appear to be stationary but inside the leaves there are juices or sap flowing, that is a 'Different Level of Reality'. Inside concrete walls atoms are moving; that is the 'alternate realm' they were referring to. Physical things that are not 'seen' are Not magical.

GLOBAL DRUG USE IN HISTORY: Egyptian mummies found with cocaine which only grew in South America, proving there was very early trade around the globe.

(Genetic memories can be triggered by psychoactive substances, see DNA section)

PAST LIVES MYTHS / REINCARNATION MYTHS & DNA

2 Big, New DNA Ideas:

1) Our DNA / Genes Are Changing Every Minute, Every Day !

2) We Have In Our Genetic Code Our Ancestors DNA Code Which Includes All the Big Events That Impressed into Them !

Every cell & molecule adapts / changes a small amount with every experience. Everything that occurs is encoded into the DNA, the more impactful an external event is, the bigger the genetics change, small events may be barely noticed, especially over generations.

The Revolutionary Take-Away From this new DNA Information Is That We Have The Power To Change Our Core Being Every Day & therefore Change Our Future.

100 years ago they thought genes were fixed, static, but new research shows that our genes change every minute ! Complex cells like the eyes take a long time to change But They Do ! Juice !

The DNA your ancestors gave you is your base set & then you modify it every day. Remember when the govt warned about LSD changing / altering our genes ? Their facts were correct ! BUT they made it sound bad, change & adaptation is Good ! Gov't Agencies & Companies just did not want kids to see a non-corporate life view.

Your ancestors experiences became coded into their DNA and then were passed into your DNA. They are deeper in our genetic memories, harder to reach, some call it the subconscious. How to get to those memories ? Hypnosis, Psychedelics, Meditation.

BLOOD BROTHERS, KISSING, SEX are all transfers of DNA through BODY FLUIDS. Fluids on skin can be washed easily, germs / bacteria need an entry port. Exchanging blood-DNA means the other person's million years of ancestors memory coding (DNA) enters our bloodstream. Men drank tiger's blood to become fierce but it does not happen overnight. see STD section pg 67

REINCARNATION MYTHS EXPLAINED: Your parents & grandparents lives are passed to you in their sperm & egg, therefore, You are the 'Reincarnation' of Your Genetic Ancestors ! You are the current physical representation of their genes.

1) Why does the hypnotized person speak 14th century flemish? It is in their genetic code from their ancestors.
2) Why are some children advanced musicians*? It is in their genetic code from their ancestors.
3) The woman under hypnosis speaking & reading hyeroglyphics & showing them where to dig in egypt & they found the palace area she described ? Her ancestor's genes & memories past on to her ?

REINCARNATION: The common idea is souls passing from body to body but that is a misunderstanding of what the ancient wise were trying to explain. Dead bodies decay into the soil which grows new life, 'from dust unto dust', thus energy is re-incarnated. Eating food grown in the soil composed of millions of generations of deceased organisms is the ultimate recycling & reincarnation.

The above idea of reincarnation as purely DNA passed on to the children is blown apart by at least one incident; the 3yr old child who remembers the naval ship details that he died on as a past-life adult; how could the pilot's genes with the memory of his own death get into this distant child's memory ? Maybe there are souls ?

ORIGIN OF REINCARNATION ? Imagine cavepeople saw a friend die & then a baby is born; the baby may have been seen as the reincarnated friend ! Imagine cavepeople saw a shooting star & then a birth occurs the next day; this could lead to thinking that each star was a person.

the 'SOUL': If someone is scared of death then the idea of a 'soul' gives them a future to focus on. The soul idea is said to come from dreams where we think we are separate from our body. A person's energy field is a physical thing, called the aura, some people can see it. Powerful people have more physical &/or mental energy. A person's energy / warmth can stay in a room after they die, but not for long.

Lost Abilities: Brain & Physical: Brains create thought, neural impulses which are electrical processes, a physical phenomenon,we just can't see them! Brains are like radio transmitters & receivers. New research finds that all of us have untapped brain abilities but those subtle circuits have been covered up over millions of years of evolving. For better modern world survival, we developed our analytical brain matter which covers our animal cortex, suppressing it; good for society, bad for our physical senses. Notice how animals have their heightened senses, they have not become overly-analytical like us big-brain humans:

—how do birds, butterflies navigate 3,000 mile migrations ? following the electromagnetic vibrations of the spinning earth.

--how do dogs hear what humans cannot ? their senses are not covered over by the analytical cortex humans developed, animals still hear the higher sound vibrations

--how do owls catch mice at night ? They can see the infrared mice body oil trails

--why do tides happen ? the gravitational pull of the moon as it gets closer to the earth, subtle vibrations. The Moons 28 day cycle makes a Women's 28 day cycle; those are strong gravitational vibrations.

1st VS 2nd CHILD GENES: The child born when the parent is 20yrs old is given different genes then the 2nd child born when parent is 40 years old because the parent's genes changed every day since the 1st child was conceived; how much they change will vary according to the mother on a case-by-case basis.

PSYCHICS: Edgar Cayce's 10,000 verified psychic readings of patient's distant maladies, which came after his brain injury, prove there is 'some brain-wave action going on'. Many telepathic / clairvoyant people have had brain trauma, causing a brain re-wiring. Telepathic occurrences are most common among family members, indicating a DNA connection. Telepathy among strangers could be explained as distant DNA cousins, however lover's telepathy indicates a different type connection.

Nostradamus & Balik foretelling future events is explained saying that Time is circular, all events have already happened, the zen view of time as non linear. Very hard for me to think of, raised in the west, reading left to right instead of the eastern life view with no heaven/hell/creator god, horizontal writing, oral vs written ?

AKASHIC RECORD ? that all info is floating in the universe that humans can tap into for ideas ? there are energy waves but can they contain full ideas ? coming to us from space ? That sounds too strange but Nostradamus ? Vague predictions ? 3 came true of thousands ? Makes me wonder....

Earth's History: Newest archeology shows the earth keeps getting bombarded with meteors & asteroids causing worldwide floods & earth axis changes. Dinosaurs wiped out, Oyantetanbo, Gobekli Tepi, Chinese 10 Story Underground Stadiums. Dinosaur Size Plants & Grand Canyon full of water; the earth's past was more lush, greener, wetter; the earth is drying out, save water !

RELIGION & RESPONSIBILITY

Q: " Why did this Happen ? " A: " God or the gods willed it. "

Because we live socially with people we tend to see events as having a social cause, caused by someone, like God, instead of an impersonal cause like gravity or earthquakes. Many say: "The devil made me do wrong" or "God helped me win". You were the one who chose wrong or your skills earned you the win.

Our Futures Will be Better if We Take Responsibility for Our Actions & Realize Our Own Power in Our Lives.

Believing our lives are governed by outside forces or gods causes a lack of personal responsibility & that becomes a problem for society. It's easier for people to blame someone or something (gov't, etc.) for their problems instead of realizing their actions are a part of the problem. People hope or pray their god will help them, but a real solution will come from our own work on fixing problems.

Do Not Depend on a God, Do Things For Yourself !

Religions Make People Feel Better. Religions mostly came about to explain what happens after death. When earthquakes kill good people, a need for reassurance, emotional stability, creates 'reasons / myths / gods' to blame for the earthquake & some say god's anger was because of our 'evil' actions, the earthquake is our fault. Religious thought like this causes Guilt, so pay the church an indulgence.

Hell ? HELL NO ! Many children are emotionally & psychologically terrorized for their whole lives by HELL. Christianity originally did not have the concept of hell, it was a scare tactic added to catholicism later by the vatican. 'Original Sin' was added to church dogma by St. Augustine, they make this stuff up ! " Immortality is Not a concept in the Bible " -Spinoza

Christianity, Protestantism & Many Religions teach that praising oneself is prideful, a sin, that this earthly world is full of devil sin so enjoying earth's pleasures was wrong. What a shame for those people deprived of pleasure from religious teachings. Developing belief in ourselves is what all religions should work to achieve.

" The Christian emphasis on an individual soul came out their stifled political hopes (against the romans) Societal virtue was less important than individual virtue: adultery was a worse crime than taking a political bribe. "- B. Russell

WESTERN vs EASTERN View of Life:
Western: God is 'up-there' & people are his servants fighting evil for a goal of heaven. Adam 'screwed up' because of a woman & we all fell from 'grace' so we're trying to get back to grace. Life is striving for salvation. God has special people, they tell us they are special.

Eastern: Everything is Part of the Universe called god, there was no fall from grace, no mistake by man. god is Not everyWHERE, god is everyTHING. god is Not a separate entity, Life IS what they term 'god'. -J. Campbell paraphrased (I monitored his class at UCSC, watch his George Lucas produced 10 part video)

Goddess Culture VS Male Religions: In BC 30,000 there were Goddess Cultures focused on the Maternal Life-Giving Spirit, not individual achievements. **Women were revered because they gave birth & their Menstrual Cycle was thought to bring the Full Moon, ancient cave-people may have thought women controlled the Moon !** All of Nature was valued, animals, trees, etc

Northern european tribes conquered the Goddess Cooperative Cultures of sumer & crete with their male religions focus on individuals, Zeus, Yahweh, Jesus, instead of the community. Even later, Peter pushed Mary Magdalene out & the Gnostic Scriptures were banned because they advocated the inclusion of women as teachers & bishops. -R. Eisler ' The Chalice & the Blade ' PS In BC 700, girls were sent to all-girls schools (island of Lesbos) to develop their 'Goddess Nature' away from male dominance. "Mothers are central to our tribe ". -Hopis

Nature as god: " there are tribes who refuse to imprison their gods within walls or to represent them in human form lest they do outrage to their majesty; tribes who prefer to worship & revere the woods & forests of their territory, and for whom the mysterious solitudes where they adore their unseen deities seem to become identified with the Divine itself. " -Tacitus, 100yrs after Jesus

Dreams Causing Religious Myths: During dreams we feel we are traveling, doing things, which gives us the impression that we have a part of us (a soul) separate or detached from our body. Dreams are projections of the mind, they are not real, they do not happen. One in a million dreams come true, same odds as the state lottery.

AURAS are a physical phenomena caused by the circulation of the blood which causes a small electrical charge. Auras are not a hoax, they have been physically proven & photographed with special cameras. Sensitive people can see them, most of us cannot.

VISITATIONS & HALLUCINATIONS occur from sleep deprivation, fasting, chanting, drumming, drugs, ayahuasca, or alcohol are Not Real. They are just projections from our mind, possibly from our right brain which cannot speak but has thoughts, maybe from our memories, things we heard &/or imagined, nothing more than apparitions of the mind. *If a god/angel/alien gave a message to one person why would they not appear at a mass gathering/sport event to tell a larger population ? Were stories about gods coming to earth merely meteors ? ps Inter-stellar travel is not possible.*

Prayer ? Some people pray but never DO anything. If 'God' is all knowing how can our prayer change his mind & isn't asking for a change insulting him ? Thoughts do produce an electrically weak signal but Praying is not Acting. If you cannot do something physical to help, in your prayers think of specific actions to help & then communicate those ideas to someone who will ACT. *Works are Stronger than Faith, Action is better than Prayer, correct action that is, discuss your ideas & future acts with others because bad acts can come from good intentions.*

Ancient Peoples & Religious Terms: Most of the ancient world did not have a word that meant 'RELIGION'; not in Greece, or Egypt or the Far East. Life was part of the cosmos, there was no separation between daily life & the spiritual realm. Buddha is not a god, he is respected. The Tao is not a religion, it is a guide to achieving a balanced life. If you translate 'god' into eastern languages it translates as all of life, the universe, not a separate being that watches over us. We are specks of dust in the universe so Enjoy Life While You Can !

Since atoms, universal energy, are inside everything then you could change the words & call universal energy 'god' & then say god is in everything. Explaining to uneducated people about protons spinning in rocks would be hard so call it 'god' instead of 'universal energy atoms'. Plato used the word 'Energy' instead of the word god. If you think from the western / dualistic view and think of god being a 'person' / specific entity, then the universal energy concept gets confused. Mistaking that we are separate from plants & animals VS we're all made of the same star dust, meaning 'we are all one'.

All religions believe 'supernatural agents' (gods, angels, etc) created the world on purpose for us & these gods know what is true. After death we survive in an unseen realm where life's purpose is known. Rituals can provoke these 'agents' to alter the world for the better. These thoughts spring from the dreams we all experience, which seem real. -S. Atran

Atheism: *" As an Atheist you can be happy, balanced, moral & intellectually fulfilled, becoming an Atheist is a brave & splendid choice. Atheism represents a healthy independence of mind. "*
-R.Dawkins 'God Delusion'. ps Thomas Paine died disowned by the country he helped found because of his anti-christian views, except by Thomas Jefferson, the atheist. " God said: Well if Atheists don't believe in Me then I don't believe in Atheists ! " -The Simpsons

" I see little evidence of goodness in this christian god's daily acts of cruelty... I cannot revere a God of war & cancer. The Christian act of worship seems debasing rather than empowering. It involves groveling before a being who, if he exists, deserves to be denounced, not respected. Belief in Immortality comes from the egos of inferior men. Christian's heaven is revenge on those having a better time on earth.." " christianity developed as a jewish slave religion against their roman oppression with it's promise of future redemption in a magical happy place " -Mencken

" Religion is man's answer to the meaningless of events, rather than living with the oppressive burden of life's chance & necessity. 'Bad things happened because an un-seen force caused them'; a religious answer which interrupts the chain of real life events, religion is not integrated into society, it is outside.-Nilsson & Burkert

" As long as PRIESTS are considered the highest type, every other type of valuable person is devalued. Christianity is a counter-movement to the morality of strength or privilege, it is the revolt of the downtrodden, against anyone with good breeding, where the hatred of the strong became a religion...christianity first made Sexuality into something un-clean....but then reversing into a religion of love.....the pathway to life is through procreation, the Dionysian Spirit as religious expression..." " Beware the Freudian garbage in the Book of Revelations " -Nietzsche

"Fear created gods." ~Petronius & Statius

"Man created god in his likeness." ~Nietzsche

"god did not create the universe. There is no god " ~S. Hawking

"A life of guilt & fear of a god who punishes is Not what I call a meaningful life." -Hitchens

" If there is a god, we are it " -John Lennon

Some Legends or Myths are Based On Historical Facts (A Great Flood, Battle of Troy) but have details exaggerated & some are completely made-up which clouds facts. Fake Stories can still teach life lessons, aimed at children, and moral lessons to encourage or scare people into acting better.

example: A real strong Hercules lived BC 500 before Jesus but written myths said Hercules healed the sick, descended to hell, resurrected, etc, the same myths as Horace in Egypt. Hercules' myths exaggerated him, myths exaggerate the real stories' facts.

THE BURIAL SCAM because of the FEAR OF DEATH

Superstitious Peoples of History & Today

Fear of Death is the fear of this truth:

We Are Dust and into Dust We Shall Return.

Cavemen created an afterlife which helped people emotionally and gave their lives a goal. People pay religions lots of money to ensure entry to an unproven afterlife through it's made-up burial requirements.

People Believe illogical Ideas because It Is Easier To Believe than to Analyze & Debate Difficult New Ideas.

The Egyptian Pharaohs, Chinese Emperors & Mayan Kings were among the biggest chumps of the ancient world, falling for the after-life stories told to them by their priests. The priests duped the rulers with their 'after-life' stories & then robbed the graves later. Priests told rulers: "You'll need to have possessions in the after life and you can buy them from my brother." A quest for immortality became the central theme of these cultures, which morphs into ego desire and a twisted view of life and it's relationships, but enough about me ! Ha!

MUMMIES: Each of these world cultures had the same belief in mummification & the resurrection of the body. But with billions dead and not a single mummy ever haven 'risen up', how does this silly ritual continue? The Fear of Death is scary, fear of the dark too, Get Over It ! Accept that we all die, face the facts, prepare mentally and emotionally for our deaths and Enjoy Life until death comes, All of Life is Preparing to Accept Our Death.

Facing Our Death and the Passing Of Others: Yes, we are upset over the loss of a loved one but a positive attitude can also occur as we CELEBRATE the good that the deceased did as mourners do in the Caribbean & New Orleans with Music & Dancing & Rejoicing about the departed's life.

Wrong to go Too deep into a negative event: Yes, we mourn a loss but focusing on your loss is Selfish. Celebrate the Positive Parts of the deceased's life. Going deep into your pain is a negative direction, STAY OUT of the Negative Neural Pathways. Looking back & recognizing wrong choices is Good but then Move On.

What Is After Death ? 1,000,000,000 , Billions of people have died & we have a few stories of 'seeing a light' ? or seeing deceased relatives & talking to them. In our final hours as physical systems fail the chemicals released to the brain can cause hallucinations mixed with memories & desires. We should not be swayed by profiteers during the emotional time of a loved one's passing. Before a passing occurs a plan is always good & helps prepare everyone emotionally.

" Dying Proudly when it is no longer feasible to live proudly, death at the right time, carried out with lucidity & cheerfulness, surrounded by relatives & friends with a real assessment of everything that has been Achieved or Willed, a Summation of their Life - in contrast to the pathetic & horrible comedy that Christianity stages around the hour of death. " -Nietzsche (see Leary's death)

No Immortality: There is no individual immortality, the idea of our soul living on is a combination of ego, a fear of death & a negation of nature's cycle of birth-death. The ancient goddess cultures revered our natural life, nature is our home, our ' Heaven ' on earth, among our loved ones. Our individual energy does live on in atoms but more importantly in the impact we have on others.

<u>**Origin of Rituals of Sacrifices to gods & Reading Entrails:**</u>

1) Village had good crop year

2) Then a bad crop year came

3) Smart con men (selfish shamans, priests) advise people that village's bad actions have caused the need to give gods gifts to get a good crop again

4) When villagers go home the con men eat the gifts !

Reading entrails: an obvious scam to get a villager to kill one of their animals ' to see what the gods say ' & then what do they do after ? " As long as the animal is dead, Let's Eat ! "

UNSEEN FORCES: YES THERE ARE ! Sound is an unseen force. Radiation from the Sun is an unseen force. Peoples who talk of unseen forces are correct that unseen forces affect us. The Moon's gravity makes ocean waves, inside our blood too, daily & monthly.

Eulogy Guideline:

- 1) Start with a couple of emotionally touching memories

- 2) Next add a story or 2 that involves people attending & mention them by name

- 3) Next add a couple Positive, Fun Stories to get a chuckle going, ending with " We Miss (Deceased) But They Would Not Have Wanted Us To Be Gloomy, Let's Remember The Good Times & Celebrate All The Positive Things That (Deceased) Did ! "

Dying Bed or Late-Life Requests: Nice to honor the dead but No deceased relative has ever complained if a difficult request is not done. Late-Life Requests are often ideas that they never completed themselves or maybe just their way of ending on a future plan, not wanting focus on their passing itself. Arduous journeys to spread ashes ? If it is fun, do it, but arduous ? Going through deceased belongings should not be done alone & make it fun, with music. The deceased is at peace now, relaxxxxx.

" No hells on earth, No christian heaven, no communist future utopia, just people living here & now instead of in some imaginary universe. " -Huxley

Mayan Calendar, Most Accurate in the World: Think of the thousands of years, night after night the Mayans, Greeks, Chinese & others laid under the stars charting the stars movements, info handed down around night fires, on cocoa, peyote, mushrooms, mead. Mayan calendar has 20,000 year ice age cycles ! Their writings said that global calamities come at the end of these cycles & this cycle's calamity (starting 2012) would be caused by Water! Oceans Rising, Flooding ! BUT, even though they were great observers of eclipse patterns, like most ancient cultures they stupidly believed 'gods' needed human blood & sacrificed 20,000 people in one big festival week wrote the spanish priests.

MAYANS & BUDDHA: Ancient Chinese explored the americas, if they had wanted to conquer, the Central & South Americans would be Buddhists Now ! (google buddhist temples found in Grand Canyon BC)

" Death is like Stupidity, it is only painful for others. " -Gervais

MUSIC & DANCING are IMPORTANT for ALL AGES

The brain following & learning musical notes is similar neurological training as learning math and starts in the womb. Listening stimulates and learning to perform on an instrument is brain training on an even higher level. Soothing music or Stimulating music, whichever mood you want at the time. Do not let societal pressures keep you off the dance floor, move your body to the music !

" A person whose activities are accompanied by music is whole, a person whose life is unmusical has a divided mind, making music gives passions expression... " A. Bloom

**For Psychological Health, ask the Greeks,
Music should be at the Center of Education.**

" Music quiets the storm of the soul, chases away the cloud of gloom and dampens the uncontrolled tumult of frenzy " -Richards
" ...calms the savage beast..." -?

**Dancing & Singing are Great Physical Releases
Relieving Muscle Stress thereby aiding
Restful Sleep & Bringing Contentment, Happiness !**

There is a playfulness to music that is healthy for the brain as it follows along with the musical notes. Our brains get to relax from the normal thinking routine, kind of like the way a meditation relaxes our brain, but the mind following an external pattern is fun !

Singing: causes a vibration in our skull which loosens our cranial fluids, increasing cranial activity, mentally stimulating !

Concerts can be seen as giving concert-goers the same community-sharing feeling of religious gatherings in these times where organized religion has become stale with their old ideas and hymns. Concerts are a community joined by the Power of Music transforming mediocrity into ecstasy. Music also has the ability to replace sorrow, to remind us to rejoice in living!

Our nervous system receives the musical notes (sound waves) exciting neural activity which can be ecstatic. Either Acoustic Instruments with their organic music waves or the power of the amplified electrical sound, music makes the brain follow the note pattern, it occupies the mind, it keeps the mind busy, good for restless people.

Music is the oldest human activity not related to food, sex or shelter. 40,000 Year Old Flutes have been found, one wood, one Ivory, to carve an ivory flute takes a lot of time ! Where did Music come from ? the Birds.

Do Not embarrass your children: NO clarinets, violins or wind instruments. (recording studio sign: ' Use an accordion, go to Jail ! ' (see Childhood section pg 64)

" The music seemed to be physically connected with my body, as if it was the amplification of the beat of my blood vessels or the neurons of my brain. " - D. Angsten

Traveling while listening to music: it enhances the scenery. " the farther out in the world I am the better music sounds; as epic scenery unfolds in front of me, with my soundtrack, the world becomes a massive wide shot " -H. Rollins

" ...as a Beautiful Melody Comes From a Piano, Our Most Profound Thoughts are Created By Our Brains " Maugham

POSITIVE THOUGHTS Can Lead to NEGATIVE RESULTS !

" It Will All Work Out For The Best ! " - from a Dreamer

"Everything Happens For a Reason" - Not always a good reason

If Thoughts Contain Wrong Ideas, They Will Lead To Wrong Actions & Bad Results !

Just because someone has a Positive attitude it does not mean they are doing Good. The damage done by 'supposed' positive actions has led to many problems because they were misguided through a lack of correct information. (Crusaders killing Muslims ?)

You Cannot Trust Family Or Friends Or Associates To Tell You That Your Idea Is Wrong, get Unbiased Advice.

Even trained psychiatrists cannot be trusted to tell you that you are wrong because their primary goal is to keep the patient coming back for years. We are all taught that to criticize is not nice. Even strangers will not tell you anything critical to your face for fear of retaliation. Life is busy, crowded & complicated, people with experience save us time & money. Get Outside Professional Opinions, Advice & Guidance.

WRONG: **" You Can Do Anything if You Try Hard !"** We all have limitations; physical, vocally, mentally. This 'cheerleading' advice causes problems as people learn that they can Not do everything. The idea that these do-gooders want to instill is that **it is good to try for what you want.** But what they instead instill is unrealistic expectations because children are told they can do anything !

We equate POSITIVE with doing good, but:

-a missionary thinks good is changing local tribes customs

-a thief can have a positive view of adjusting financial inequality

-You can have a Positive Attitude as you drink poison (sodas ?)

" Something Good Will Come Out of It " Nice to Hear but Can Lead to Inactivity through a made-up positive view. Good may be found but good is not always there, it's a placebo phrase. How about: " Let's see if something good comes out of this but if not hopefully we'll learn not to do this again ! "

These pleasant sounding proverbs are delusional. A Volcanic destruction of a village of nice people did Not work out Best & there was No Reason for it ! You can make up all kinds of explanations or conditions (see MAKING THINGS UP section):
False Idea: maybe volcanic victims were bad people ?
False Idea: some kind of good outcome happened (a baby lived ?)

We can learn a lesson from negative events but putting a positive spin on the negative event is trying to cover it up with a positive thought. Do Not cover up the negative event, Face It, acknowledge it & your role in it & vow to try not to make the same mistake again !

KARMA Krap-Ola: Karma's Premise is not about specific actions. Karma is a general energy concept, not tied to every specific bad action. The concept is referring to the negative energy of a bad action, the guilt, the 2nd guessing, someone eventually finding out, BUT, none of that may Happen ! Unfortunately, Good Things Can Happen to Bad People.
KARMA NOT WORKING: the american 'robber barons'; they got away with killing their workers, poisoning rivers, etc and lived to be rich & old. Let's try to make sure the bad folks do not get away with bad things, that would make us 'Karma-Kops' ! ha !

<u>Fad Foods Part 2</u>, <u>Fad Cures, Fad Diets</u>

These are quick comments, this whole book covers these issues.

-ACCUPUNCTURE ? This is used in china for serious surgeries. In rich cities this has become a fad foisted on gullible people; ACCUPRESSURE / MASSAGE touches the same energy points & is much less invasive, more relaxing & healing.

-BONE JUICE ? sure, it has minerals but also the toxins the animal could not eliminate, what a scam.

-BEE POLLEN / ROYAL JELLY ? Honey is a wonderful substance, pollen & jelly are fads with exaggerated facts for profit.

-AFIB: How many catchy names are they going to come up with to scare people to buy pills ? Heart Problems ? See CHEESE section

-MALE SEX PILLS: Side Effects show up later. See Sex section.

-HEALTH BOOKS / DIET BOOKS; Most Nutrition Books are funded by dairy or meat corporations. Not this one ! $ Billions have been spent by the Dairy Lobby to convince people that Milk, Cheese & Eggs are healthy to consume. Dairy ok in small quantities but Dairy clogs arteries causing heart attacks.

-SLEEP APNEA; WHAT A SCAM ! Yes, sleep patterns can be interrupted by breathing disruptions; we cough, we may hold our breath during a dream; this does not mean we have a condition that needs a breathing machine !

-HEART MEDICATION / BLOOD THINNERS: Fatty, greasy foods make thick blood that the heart cannot pump easily. Pill-Doctors prescribe these pills to speed up the entire system & heart, (doctors get a small kickback for every pill sold) Vegetables make more watery blood so blood pumps easier. Heart Pills Side Effects: New research shows brain damage from these pills, google CNN.

-RAW: Of course many raw vegetables are great, HOWEVER, this 70-90% RAW FAD does not give busy people the 'Heat' needed for modern busy life. Cooked Foods Also Gave Homo Sapiens Larger Brains ! much more pg 144

-CANCER & DRUG ADDICTION TREATMENT CENTERS:
Preying on the fearful & uneducated. see Cancer & Addiction sections pages 56 & 102.

-ASPIRIN REGIMEN ? People eat a high-fat diet & want aspirin to thin their fatty blood ? Pills build up internally & have side-effects. Aspirin is for when you have mild pain, not daily consumption.

-MAKEUP OBSESSION: " I cannot go out of the house without my makeup face " -Revlon brainwashed you to think that. The natural beauty of women gets covered with powder. The 'over-powdered' look is unattractive no matter what your girlfriends say, it is a manifestation of psychological & emotional insecurity.

Yes, eyes look more alluring with some mascara, but magazines make women think you look 'unfinished' without makeup, that is brainwashing. Men are brainwashed by magazines also, their tastes need to be re-trained.

A 'Pretty Face' comes from bone structure, Pretty Faces can have mud on them & they are still Pretty ! Not everyone may be called 'pretty' by the standards of the day or your region but there is Beauty in Every Face, Be Proud of Your Individual, Unique Natural Feminine Beauty & Never Feel Ashamed that You Don't have society's Makeup On !

Makeup is overused by the Insecure.

-SUN POWER: Living things evolved in Sun Light ! Indoor living has made people lose their billion year connection to the Power & Necessity of the Sun, it gives us vitamins that cannot be duplicated in a lab. Some people have become so mole-like, the sun's power bothers them, expose yourself gradually but get back to being a normal Sun-Loving Animal. All ancient cultures worshipped the Sun, until paul became the money collector for christianity. (we say worshipped, how about Respected ? Revered ?)

-MY doctor, MY therapist, MY hair stylist: This is often said with a possessive attitude coming from a desire to be attached, or to own, which comes from an insecure place. Insecurity Solution: Learn to Love Yourself from Doing Good Works so that you do not need external validation, although it is nice. " the stylist I go to, he is Not mine " you don't own him / her.

-EYE DROPS: Yes, our eyes can get dry but ADDING MAN-MADE CHEMICALS TO OUR MILLION YEAR DESIGNED EYES has side-effects. Try wetting with ordinary water before using chemical eye solutions. NEW EYE FACTS: Eyes can Improve ! Old science said eyes & genes do not change, better tests show they do change, mostly slowly but can change fast, depending. Avoid hard liquor and dairy products to keep our vision from 'clouding up'.

-ENEMAS ? for Health ?? Shoving an external anything up there & stretching tissues; bad. See SEX section for more anal advice.

-WIRELESS DEVICES: Why receive more brain microwaves vs using a little cord ? CNN reports Brain Damage 2019

-CALORIES: A made-up system by the FDA in 1950 to confuse the public into putting fatty meats & dairy in the same calorie system as brown rice, vegetables, beans, nuts, fruits & all the healthy foods.

-ZERO CALORIES / NO SUGAR: Bull Crap ! These claims are absurd. Use your logic, no matter what a paid scientist says these claims of zero calories are physically impossible.

-SKIM MILK / NON-FAT: yes these contain less clogging fat but it is still animal milk made from their fatty blood which are not human genetics, become a Cow ! On my granola, cereal or Oatmeal I switched to soy milk, then rice milk, then apple juice. The tongue's taste buds get trained early BUT can be un-trained & will get used to whatever we are exposed to, it takes time, but every bite changes us !

-EGGS, CHEESE & MILK for Adults who have Slower Metabolisms ?? Come On, Think ! Eggs have the same heavy viscosity or thickness as motor oil. See CHEESE MYTHS pg 21&13

-PSORIASIS / RASHES: The skin is an organ of Elimination of Toxins, skin ruptures are the body throwing off the toxins you are eating ! Cure: Stop eating crap food, cut down on grease, sugar & chocolate. See RASHES section pg 37

-NARCOLEPSY ? Modern Busy Life makes Us All Exhausted; REST MORE ! NAPS ! All animals take naps & all world cultures except the USA ! Do not take pills with Long-Term Side-Effects. See INSOMNIA section

-BOTOX for Migraines: Absurd ! Do Not inject pig fat that later dissolves into your brain ! See MIGRAINES page 32

-HIV PILL: Scam ! Trying to get people to take a daily preventative pill, preying on people's confusion & fear. See HIV-AIDS page 54

-CAYENNE / GINGER: These are powerful herbs used to 'blow out' clogged intestines or arteries, 'blow out' fatty deposits. Taking these as on a regular basis will cause an imbalance in your system as you have to use up your other minerals to counter-balance these powerful agents.

-CLAY has minerals, but don't eat it ! money, money, money...

-YOGURT: yes, it's bacteria gives digestive help but the cow fat clogs. There are many probiotic foods that aid digestion without dairy fat: pickles, salad, sauerkraut, miso soup. see Cheese Myths in Osteoporosis section pg 13.

-PROTEIN MYTH: Excess protein causes excess cell growth (cysts, cancer). Meat Companies have distorted this subject for their profit. (see Protein Excess section)

-TELEVISION DRUGS ? why is every other tv ad about drugs ? Because they make a fortune selling pills ! all with side effects that take 20 years to discover after the patients have liver or kidney problems. Eat vegetables & oatmeal for 2 weeks & watch how you feel better !

-ORGANIC: of course this is better but not to obsess over. Pesticides are everywhere, even in the water that feeds onto Organic Farms so it's never going to be perfect, we just try.

-BEE VENOM FACIAL: newest form of Idiocy

-Flu Shots: Potentially Dangerous. Viruses mutate every day BUT so does our Immune System ! We create new anti-bodies to combat the new strains that every day enter our nose & mouth. Injecting a foreign virus in our system, a flu shot, can overwhelm our Immune System & make you sicker. Flu Shots are a big money program from the Pharmaceutical Companies & drugstores preying on the scared & uninformed.

FAD FOODS, Extended Subjects:

RAW: CONTINUED: A 70-90% RAW FOOD DIET is not healthy for busy, city people, we need the fire energy of cooked foods. Homo Sapiens received extra brain energy from fire 'breaking down' food so we got more nutrients with less stomach juices used; Cooked Foods Gave Us Larger Brains ! Cooking food made our modern genetics.

Yes, cooking takes out some vitamins BUT, the stomach cannot get the full nutrients from many Raw Foods because their fiber is too hard to break down. Sprouted seeds & immature plants (wheatgrass) are Not how our ancestors consumed these foods for the last 2 Million Years Since We Learned to Cook ! Our system does not fully metabolize sprouted grains & beans, it does not extract all the proper nutrients. Grains, Beans & Squashes & some vegetables need to be cooked.

-VITAMIN PILLS, SHAKES, POWDERS: CONTINUED: If we are taking vitamin pills our system thinks: " I'm getting the vitamin from a pill so why should I make this vitamin internally anymore ? " So our bodies shut down our natural vitamin production.

People: " the soil is depleted so I take vitamins "

Jon: " That issue is exaggerated by The Vitamin Industry. The vitamin pill, the extreme dosage boost, with negative side effects, is unhealthy. Fresh vegetable juices flood us with fresh nutrients, do not buy old vitamin pill dust. "

the uneducated: " but Jon, I felt a boost after taking the vitamin pill "

Jon: " Yes, that boost was the overdose. Pay attention & you will notice the 'come down', you'll feel more tired and depleted later, & then you'll take another without re-fueling & resting properly.

MISO SOUP HEALS RADIATION POISONING: In Japan, traditional families drink Miso before Every Meal to put fresh, live bacteria in their intestines to increase food digestion & absorption (hot or cold). Do Not boil miso, it kills the bacteria. If you make Miso Soup too salty it will make you drink too much water to counterbalance the salt; Miso Soup should be pleasantly, mildly salty. 50 Years of post atomic bomb research has shown conclusively that Miso cleans cells of radiation also !

GREAT FADS !! KALE & JUICES: Dark Green Leafy Vegetables are 2nd in importance to Grains in human diets. All Greens; Spinach, Collard Greens, Green Chard, Mustard Greens. Cook them till they are not bitter (taste as you cook) & put salad dressings on them to taste good. Juices are Not how our million-year digestive system received vitamins But since we eat so much junk / fast food, drinking juices can overcome some of the bad we do to our bodies.

Fresh Juices give our intestines & organs not only vitamins & minerals but also enzymes & other live ingredients to aid digestion. Do not pasteurize juices or miso. Juices' vitamins deteriorate quickly so drink them fast after they are juiced.

Juice Ingredients I like best Containing Soil Water w/ Minerals & Vitamins & Chlorophyl:

-Cucumber
-Celery
-Kale
-Spinach
-Beet   (strong minerals & sugar to sweeten the juice)

Can we drink too much Juices ? Yes. Moderation.

-SKIN CANCER SCARE EXAGERRATED: CONTINUED:

Cosmetic companies have paid scientists to exaggerate skin cancer scares causing a neurotic fear of sunlight. Yes, too much sun's rays burn BUT humans NEED some sunlight to have a fully healthy system, at least 15 minutes / day of pleasant sun.

Excessive sugar in the blood causes sugar cells near the skin surface to burn (freckles) but the problem is excessive sugar, not excessive sun. Yes, use sun block for strong sun exposure but no need to be neurotic about normal sun exposure. Skin cancer stories are exaggerated in the media purposely paid for by cosmetic companies. Of course outdoors workers will get bigger percentage of skin problems but that's their fault for excessive exposure. For normal people, get some of sun's vitamins & energy,

Everyone Looks Healthier With Some SunTan !

-1925 Quack Cures ? " ...thyroid extract, adrenaline, thymin, pituitrin, insulin with pick-me-ups of hormone stimulants, blood being fortified with antibodies against infections by innoculations or vaccinations of infected bacteria and serum from Infected Animals, and fortified against old age by surgical extirpation of the reproductive ducts or weekly doses of monkey gland.." -George Bernard Shaw, 1925 - Sound Familiar ?

<u>SUMMARY</u>

I wrote these pages originally in emails to friends & associates in response to their medical questions & health issues. I'm trying to help people get healthier without Pills & Surgeries because so many people are hurt by wrong information & manipulated by profit motives.

- Before Taking Pills Or Surgery, Try Changing Your Diet For A Few Weeks & Juice of Fresh Vegetables Every Day to flush out toxins.

- For Best Brain Functioning, Eat Fresh-Cooked Whole Grains Daily, Oatmeal Or Brown Rice, Easy !

It is NOT about being perfect because We All Love PIZZA ! We Love Junk Food but balance them with Fresh Foods.

Don't be a member of the 'FEAR CULTURE' that makes people think "Everything is Attacking Us ! ". Profit-driven companies want us to be scared & uninformed so we buy their cures & pills. TV commercials repeated over & over with wrong info can make you think their wrong ideas are good & they call 'chicken soup' 'witch's work' or 'quaint peasant folk wisdom'.

You Can Make Tomorrow & the Rest of Your Life Better, little by little, one small change at a time.

The Quality of Our Modern Lives is the Best They Have Ever Been in Human History, ENJOY IT !!

In Closing: I hope the natural, logical ideas in this book will be useful to the sufferers of the medical & psychological conditions discussed; I look forward to future discussions. I have shared ideas I learned from many great teachers: Domhoff, Duesberg, Kushi & Schaar to name a few of my favorites. I have received a lot of feedback about the positive life changes people have experienced from implementing the simple, natural ideas I've explained here. I've lived all this advice & I hope these ideas will bring Health to You !

Table Of Contents By CATEGORY:

1 *Alzheimer's Helped by Eating Oatmeal & All Whole Grains !*

2 **Women's Sections & Men's**

3 **Brain Nutrition & Healthy Thoughts**

4 **AIDS Myths, Cancer Myths & The Immune System**

5 **Fad Foods, Fad Diets & Fad Cures**

6 **Parenting**

7 **Reincarnation Myths / Past Lives Myths & DNA**

8 **General Health Topics**

2) Women's Sections & Men's:

Osteoporosis, Arthritis, Milk & Calcium Myths

Cheese, Yogurt Vs Avocados, Nuts: Animal Vs Vegetable Fats

The 28 Day Lunar Cycle / Birth Control

Menstruation Without Pain / Ovulation Cycles

Breast Feeding & The AIDS Connection To Our Immune System

Yoga & Meditation: Missing The Point

Masculinization Of Women & The Feminization Of Men

Aids & Cancer Myths & The Immune System

<u>Table Of Contents By CATEGORY:</u>

3) Brain Nutrition & Healthy Thoughts:

Depression & Suicidal Thoughts Stopped !

Brain Food; It's Not Fish / Do Not Eat Shellfish

Bi-polar / Autism / Dyslexia / Hyperactivity

Sex Addiction / Love Addiction: Bull Crap !

Alcoholism & Drug Addiction: Bull Crap 2 !

Perfectionists / Tough Guys / Asking For Help

Sick ? For Attention ?

Happy ? You Should Be !

Alzheimer's & Dementia Helped by Eating Whole Grains

4) AIDS MYTHS, CANCER MYTHS & THE IMMUNE SYSTEM:

STDs: A Logical Approach

Vaccinations / Flu Shots & The Immune System

5) Fad Foods, Fad Diets & FAD CURES:

Fad Foods 2 Continued

Cheese, Yogurt Vs Avocados, Nuts: Animal Vs Vegetable Fats

Protein Excess

Cheapest Vitamins & Minerals ? You're Wrong

6) PARENTING:

Children's Brain Development Ideas / Dyslexia

Living Your Life Through Your Child; Who's In Charge ?

Breast Feeding & The Aids Connection To The Immune System

Bi-polar / Autism / Dyslexia / Hyperactivity

7) PAST LIVES MYTHS / REINCARNATION MYTHS & DNA

8) GENERAL HEALTH TOPICS:

Healthy ? Cold, Flu, Strep...

Prostate and Urinary Fallacies

Sore Throat ? Migranes, Rashes: Gone !

Vaccinations / Flu Shots & The Immune System

STDs: A Logical Approach

Chiropractic Can Be Dangerous / Injuries Best Treatment

Table of Contents ALPHABETICALLY:

ALZHEIMER'S & DEMENTIA Helped by Eating Oatmeal & All Whole Grains

AIDS & CANCER MYTHS & the IMMUNE SYSTEM

Bi-Polar / AUTISM / DYSLEXIA / HYPERACTIVITY

Brain Food; It's Not Fish / Do Not Eat Shellfish

BREAST FEEDING & the AIDS Connection to the IMMUNE SYSTEM

Cheese VS Nuts; Animal FAT VS Vegetable FAT ?

Diabetes: We All Eat Too Much Sugar

Depression & Suicidal Thoughts Stopped !

HEALTHY ? Cold, Flu, Strep...

Fad Foods, Fad Diets, Fad Cures

Gluten Explained

insomnia / Night-Shift Accidents

Injuries / Chiropractic Can Damage

MASCULINE WOMEN & feminine men

Menstruation Without Pain / Birth Control / Ovulation

Osteoporosis, Arthritis / Milk & Calcium Myths

PARENTING / ABANDONMENT / Kid's DISCIPLINE

Prostate & Urinary Fallacies

PROTEIN EXCESS

SORE THROAT ? Migraines, Rashes: Cured for Life !

STDs: A Logical Approach / Infections

Best Vitamins & Minerals ? You're Wrong

VACCINATIONS, FLU SHOTS & Immune System

Jon Flanagan studied these disciplines with many
Internationally Renowned Professors including M. Domhoff,
J. Schaar & P. Duesberg:

- Neurophysiology
- Nutrition
- Psychology
- Holistic Health
- International Politics and Medicine

Attended:

- Univ. Calif. Berkeley
- UCLA
- UCSC

Published Internationally
© Jon Flanagan 2015 – 2020

<u>WARNINGS about this book:</u>

**If you get upset when your ideas are questioned, please do Not read this book.
I am Not trying to offend anyone.**

I am presenting ideas which some may see as controversial but also I am questioning &/or criticizing many mainstream, commonly held ideas, especially those that are being shown to cause negative consequences.

MARSHALL McCLUHAN Formatting *? modern grammar ?*

" ..CAPITALIZATION Hypnotizes the reader.." - Orwell

SHORT SECTIONS: I am trying to explain complex ideas using common sense language & I've kept my explanations short for easy 'digestion'. However, I am not dismissing Complex Subjects lightly that could need more explanation & discussion; I'm just trying to open the ' Doors TO Perception '... Hey !

GENERALIZATIONS: There are many generalizations in this book. If over 60% of cases exhibit a pattern then that majority is what we generalize from. There are always exceptions to the majority but arguing the exceptions slows down what we learn from the majority (see PERFECTIONISTS section)

DUPLICATE PARAGRAPHS: I have placed especially important ideas under 2 different headings so they would not be missed; I memorized ideas by reading them 3X's. (The Iron & Oxygen from Chlorophyl process took me 5X's to memorize but my teachers did not explain it as succinctly as I have here, Ha !)

Alzheimer's Prevented & Helped By Eating OATMEAL or BROWN RICE & All Whole Grains !

" Poor Diet causes ALZHEIMER's Memory Loss ! " - UCLA Medical Ctr

- Brain 'Diseases' Have Increased Dramatically from eating sugar-cereals & junk foods.

- FLOUR Clogs Brains, Oatmeal & Brown Rice does Not.

- BRAINS need the B-COMPLEX of Vitamins found in Fresh-Cooked Brown Rice, Oatmeal & All Whole Grains.

- Vitamin B Pills are dead vitamins

Meat, Cheese, Fish & Eggs have protein, fat and nutrients that the brain uses for upkeep but **Nervous System Communications depend on the B-Complex of Vitamins found in Whole Grains.**

White Flour contains Bleach ! We love Flour: Pasta, Bread & Pizza but try to eat them with Whole Grain Flour which still has the Outer Shell which is where the B-Complex of Vitamins are, the Brain Nutrients. Even whole-grain flour clogs our systems, moderation. Try to eat your grains without them being ground-up.

For a Better Brain, Eat Oatmeal Every Day !

PROTEIN in Grains: 17% in Barley. 10K & Triathlon's Winners have been Vegetarians eating Grains & Beans for Power. Grains have all the Protein Humans Need, Beans add more. Ignore the Fake protein-scare reports from meat companies.

If our Brain's Neurons & Neurotransmitters are made from processed foods they do not work as well & degenerate faster, eating bad food is like putting bad gasoline in your car engine.

VITAMIN PILLS are Old Vitamins. The Vitamin B Pill or Shot from a doctor for nervous system disorders, mental confusion or a boost is distilled from Whole Grains. Eat Oatmeal or Brown Rice or any Whole Grain & skip the doctor's pills & shots which are old, pulverized vitamins.

Whole Grain Flour or Bread is better than White but is still processed, probably with chemicals & old. Ground-Up foods lose their vitality quickly, their life force, their atomic spin. Our ancestors cooked whole grains fresh every day for 13,000 years & we went from being food gatherers to building Pyramids !

Whole Grains are a carbohydrate, a complex sugar, that we convert into glycogen for energy storage. Glycogen also helps us digest our food. Eating Whole Grains on a daily basis keeps our brain fueled with glycogen, running smoothly on a steady stream of energy so we can Think Clearly, Be Calm & Content, Happy !

White Flour & White Rice do Not contain the Brain Nutrients, the B-Complex of Vitamins which are in the Husk, which is lost when Grain is processed into Flour & Bleached & Sugared.

PLAQUE on the Brain: Gunky Plaque forms on our teeth & arteries & Our Brain Connections, especially from Flour & Cheese. Vegetables & Fruits leave ZERO plaque & they Clean Plaque with their roughage !

Old, Dead Flour: After grains are ground up the nutrient value / life force starts decaying. Stored in a warehouse, shipped to another warehouse; by the time it gets to you the nutrients are dead / minimal & then they form a 'paper-mache' like sludge in your intestines.

**Grain Power increased Brain Power,
Eating Grains lead to Civilization !**

13,000 years ago the first civilizations, Mesopotamia and China, planted the first Rice and Barley fields & then developed writing, advanced civilization. We were cave people then after growing grains we became the builders of Pyramids all over the world. ps Written records found saying Fermented Barley Beer was how the pyramid builders were paid !
fun fact: Chinese emperors were too fat & lazy to chew brown rice & had the servants remove the hull / shell to make white rice.

Forgetting Details IS NOT A Sign Of Brain Problems: As our brains are filled with new info, less important info becomes out of use & harder to recall, that is NOT a sign of brain trouble. You & yours will know when you have real brain problems !

MEMORIES CHANGING ALL THE TIME ? 2018 neurophysiology research showed that our memories do not stay the same, each time we remember an event we can add new details to the memory that were not originally there. HOWEVER, maybe the people in the above experiments had poorly functioning brains from deficient B-Complex. I suggest more specific testing with Fresh Whole Grains for 3 months & then let's check their memories again.

" A memory is a bond; a loving memory is twice as strong. " -Sweig

Old People Wisdom ? Stupid / Dumb: Wisdom does Not always come with age. If a person lives a long life it does not mean they are wise; they may be lucky or never did much. Experience alone does not mean the person learned the best or correct lessons. People often learn a wrong lesson from an experience; example; enjoying a short-term gain but not perceiving the long-term problems; Like Health Problems from Eating Junk Food ! Experience with Intelligence gives Knowledge & Wisdom. Stupid or Dumb people are Not bad people, their brains are just not processing as well as others. There are many dumb old people, don't be one of them, eat Grains for Your Brain !

Trivia OR Knowledge: Knowing details does Not mean a person understands the purpose. Trivia has little value compared to having Knowledge. You cannot fix problems or improve something without an understanding of the purpose or function. " A genius is a person who can see farther and deeper into subjects and can act (on those observations) " -George B. Shaw

Junk Food Eaters Who Are Not Sick ?? Confusion Explained: How long does it take for a healthy body to deteriorate from Junk Food ? You can exercise & look good on the outside but why do fit-looking 50yr olds have heart attacks ? Arteries clogged with fats & junk foods. A child may go 60 years on good genetics even while eating junk food but then their kids would be given junk food genes.

We now have the great-grandchildren of the 1st junk food generations. Look at our modern society to see their health & mental stability. A person cannot eat junk food & stay healthy. If your Brain is getting only Junk Food it will not work at it's best. Just because a mind can compute details does not mean it is balanced, with empathy, without negative thoughts & with an understanding of our place in our community; Being Happy !

One-Minute Oatmeal is the easiest way to get B-Complex daily.
- 5 minute Oatmeal has better quality B-Complex Vitamins.
- 30 minute Oatmeal, 50 minute Brown Rice & All Grains has Best Quality.
- White Rice is better than No rice, try for less chemicals.

Our Ancestors and their Animals built this Country Eating Oatmeal & Oats !

Make Healthy Food Taste Good with Sauces & Dressings: Flavor your food with whatever you like to make the healthy food Taste Good ! Boil Oatmeal in apple juice and boil Brown Rice in tomato sauce or whatever flavors you like ! Some point out: " the sauces have oils & additives ". That is too small a concern;

" A Spoonful Of Sauces Helps The Grains Go Down ! "

The GRAIN DEBATE:

2 BOOKS THAT OTHER DOCTORS
SAY HAVE WRONG IDEAS:

' GRAIN BRAIN ' & ' WHEAT BELLY ' should be named:

' FLOUR Brain ' & ' FLOUR Belly '

These books warn about grains but their warning should be about
FLOUR WITH CHEMICALS & WHITE RICE that has been
bleached with chemicals & sugar added.

Their research HAS NOT included FRESH WHOLE GRAINS:
Brown Rice, Barley, Wheat, Millet, Oatmeal, Corn, etc.

They also wrongly recommend eating Animal's Organs, Clams &
Eggs, the Big 3 Heart Attack Foods ! This is misguided advice.

Another ANTI-GRAIN IDEA currently: CAVITIES: Some now say
after grain cultivation, 13,000. yrs ago, teeth fossils show more
decay, which they attribute to the starch in grains.
1) can the few examples they found cover everyone ?
2) During that time we went from caves to growing grains, farming,
built pyramids & civilization so if they are right I say a few cavities
was worth it.
3) this is the time of distilled alcohol, could alcohol have led to tooth
decay & it was not barley but barley beer that caused decay ?

Impossible Burger / Beyond Meat: ALL CHEMICALS !

New Ideas Presented in this Book:

- **Breast Feeding Prevents AIDS, HIV & Immune System Deficiencies.**

- **Brain Communication & Functions Improved by the B-Complex from Fresh Whole Grains, Not pills.**

- **DNA / GENES Update Daily & Contain Our Ancestor's Individual Genetic DNA Coding.**

www.ingramcontent.com/pod-product-compliance
Lightning Source LLC
Chambersburg PA
CBHW031228250726

48655CB00005B/1850